The
Fearless
Caregiver

The Fearless Caregiver

How to Get the Best Care for Your Loved One and Still Have a Life of Your Own

Gary Barg

Editor-in-Chief, *Today's Caregiver Magazine*

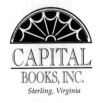

CAPITAL
BOOKS, INC.
Sterling, Virginia

First paperback edition 2003

Capital Books, Inc.
P.O. Box 605
Herndon, Virginia 20172-0605

Library of Congress Cataloging-in-Publication Data

The fearless caregiver : how to get the best care for your loved one and still have a life of your own / Gary Barg, editor. — Pbk. ed.
     p. cm.
  ISBN 1-931868-56-5
    1. Caregivers—Popular works. I. Barg, Gary. II. Title.

RA645.3.F437   2003
362.1—dc21

                                                        2003012212

Printed in the United States of America on acid-free paper that meets the American National Standards Institute Z39-48 Standard.

Designed by Pen & Palette Unlimited

First Edition

10 9 8 7 6 5 4 3 2

3 42.1
FCa
v1

Contents

Acknowledgments

For my mother, Monica Weiss Barg, whose love of family is the heart and soul of everything we do.

I have been blessed since beginning on this journey in working with some of the best people with the biggest hearts who have supported me with their love, time, and encouragement. That of course includes my mom, my brother Steven, my sister Linda Manzini and family, Chris Andaya, Rick Harris, my editor and dear friend Nancy Schonwalter, creative director Adnan Razack, Elaine, Monica, Rona, Susan, Suzanne and Steve, Connie, Judy, Terry, Sonja and Mike, Les and Melissa. Thanks to our friends at Internet.com, Alan Meckler and Howard Neuthaler.

I would also like to thank Kathleen, Jeanne, Dorothy, and Noemi at Capital Books, Inc. as well as our former editors, Salha Mishaan and Kate Murphy, R.N. To all of those others who have supported us these past seven years and to all caregivers, past, present, and future, go the thanks of a grateful author. When I think about the contribution made by the writers who have shared their wisdom with us, I am at a loss for words. To me, every article is pure poetry.

Most important of all, to my father, Robert Barg, and my grandfather, Joseph Weiss: We miss you both very much and think of you daily. "This one's for the both of you."

The Contributors

Christian Andaya, R.P.T. has been a professional caregiver and physical therapist for seven years. He has worked in outpatient services, rehabilitation hospitals, nursing homes, and home health agencies. He can be reached at <u>Chris@ caregiver.com</u>.

Gary Barg is the founder and editor-in-chief of *Today's Caregiver Magazine* and <u>www.caregiver.com</u>, which were founded in 1995. He is a recognized expert in the field of family caregiving and has appeared on NBC's *Today Show* and in interviews with *American Health for Women, The Miami Herald, Investor's Business Daily,* and other major publications. He has been a keynote speaker at the International Senior Fair, Huntington's Disease Society of America's annual conference, the Successful Aging Conference and master of ceremonies at "Sharing Wisdom," the national Caregivers Conference, for the past three years.

Monica Weiss Barg is executive editor of *Today's Caregiver Magazine* and has been a caregiver for her husband, stepmother, and father.

Jennifer Buckley is a staff writer for *Today's Caregiver Magazine* and an experienced family caregiver.

Louise K. Center, L.C.S.W. has been in private practice for over 15 years in South Florida. Ms. Center has a B.A. in psychology (University of Miami, 1965) and M.S.W. (Florida

International University, 1991). Ms. Center facilitates personal growth groups for seniors over sixty, bereavement groups, the "sandwich generation" (adults with aging family and responsibilities in their own families and jobs), peer relationships in later years, and illness in the family. She founded Senior Lifeline (seniorlifeline@aol.com) with Jennifer Kay.

Kim Champion graduated Magna Cum Laude from Florida State University in 1982. In 1993, she founded her own agency, Champion Home Health Care, Inc. With the help of her husband, Richard Stewart, the agency expanded to include licensee offices. Kim has one daughter, Alexandra, and two stepchildren, Mark and Christine.

Pamela R. Clayton, a playwright, poet, and writing teacher, along with her three sisters, has been caring for her mother since 1993. Everyone is doing well, all things considered. Pamela can be contacted by email at rdclayt@ banet.net.

Paul Dammann was born in Melbourne, Florida, and lives in Miami with his wife, Jackie, and daughters, Laura and Holly. Although, by profession, he is an oceanographer, his poetry allows him to express his innermost feelings in a way that gives both joy and understanding to those in need of a kind word.

David Dancu, N.D., J.D. is a naturopath/homeopath with twelve years' experience in assisting the body to find its own means of healing and recovery. He is the author of *Homeopathic Vibrations: A Guide for Natural Healing* (Sunshine Press, 1996) and *Natural Health Essentials.* He can be reached at www.naturalhealthessentials.com.

Margie Davis is the author of *The Healing Way: A Journal for Cancer Survivors.* She conducts a course for writers called "Writing for Personal Caregivers." She may be reached at margie@writingtoheal.com.

Douglas Eisenstark, L.Ac., is a graduate of Emperor's College, where he earned a Masters of Traditional Oriental Medicine, and maintains a private practice in acupuncture and herbology in Los Angeles, California. He can be contacted through his Web site, www.Taiqi.com or by email at douglas@taiqi.com.

Naomi Feil, M.S., A.C.S.W. is the creator of Validation Therapy. She began Validation in 1963 in response to her dissatisfaction with traditional methods of working with the severely disoriented person. She can be reached at http://www.vfvalidation.org/.

Carole Fiedler has exclusively represented the needs of the insured (the seller or/and viator) since 1992 and formed Fiedler Financial in 1994. She is considered an expert in the field of viatical and life settlements. Currently licensed in nine states and representing people nationwide, Ms. Fiedler is a strong advocate for regulation and consumer protections. For more information: www.FiedlerFinancial.com or (800) 905-0114.

Camilla Hewson Flintermann is a caregiver for her husband, Peter, who was diagnosed with Parkinson's in 1989. Camilla runs the CARE list for caregivers of people with Parkinson's, a "virtual support group" with 350+ members worldwide. A retired counselor, she is devoted to three grandchildren and one cat.

Mitchell J. Ghen, M.P.S., D.O., Ph.D. is a nationally renowned speaker and alternative medicine physician. He holds a doctorate in alternative medicine and psychoneuroimmunology, and a rabbinical degree.

Rabbi Saul Goldman is Spiritual Leader of Congregation Aliyah in Palm Air (Pompano Beach), Florida. He has been published in medical and theological journals on the relationship between religion and medicine. He serves as volunteer chaplain at several hospitals and nursing homes as well as on the ethics committee of several hospitals.

R. Nacken Gugel, Ph.D., a specialist in geriatrics and long-term care, serves as associate dean of the College of Health Sciences at Lynn University. Dr. Gugel is an adjunct associate professor in the Department of Psychiatry and Behavioral Medicine at the University of Miami School of Medicine. She serves as director of psychological services at the Miami Jewish Home and Hospital for the Aged.

Carolyn Haynali is spokesperson and founder of the Caregivers Army, an organization dedicated to all caregivers, no matter what illness or disease they battle. She can be reached at www.caregiversarmy.com/Carolyn/Home.htm.

Dan Horter has been the executive director of The Preserve at Palm-Aire, a Cordia Senior Residence, in Pompano Beach, Florida, since 1996. Dan misses his grandmother to this day.

Sherri Issa, M.S.W., L.C.S.W., D.A.B.C.M. is professional issues editor of www.caregiver.com and *Today's Caregiver Magazine*. She is an eldercare consultant and can be reached at issamsw@aol.com.

Jennifer Kay is a licensed clinical social worker in private practice in Miami, Florida. She has written numerous articles for *Today's Caregiver Magazine* pertaining to issues of illness and bereavement. In addition to serving caregivers and those who are grieving, she also provides individual and couples therapy. She can be reached at mswkay@aol.com.

Sean Kenny has been training individuals for over a decade. Certified by the American Council on Exercise and PACE, Sean is also a member of both IDEA Fitness Professionals Organization and the National Strength and Conditioning Association. Sean is currently a nationally published author and lecturer on health and fitness. His Web site is www.anythingfitness.com.

Juli Koroly is a caregiver who spent four years in the health system as a certified nursing assistant and edited a national caregivers newsletter. This full schedule gave her a unique perspective on the role of caregiver. Her mission is to support others with whom she shares this role.

Delton Krueger does Web page creation (www.interfaithcalendar.org) and is a volunteer chaplain at Hennepin County Medical Center in Minneapolis. His background is in pastoral ministry with rural and urban United Methodist congregations.

Rabbi Rita Leonard is a Jewish liturgical composer, poet, and playwright who serves as spiritual leader and cantor for the East Hawaii Havurah.

Sandi Magadov was caregiver to her son Andrew, who died from a rare form of cancer at the age of fifteen. Through her writing she has played a supportive role in the healing process of parents coping with the devastating loss of a child.

Rita Miller-Huey, M.Ed., R.D., L.D. is a registered dietitian and licensed nutritionist bringing personalized, convenient nutrition education and counseling to individuals and groups. She can be reached by email at HealthDynamics @ix.netcom.com.

Catherine Murphy, R.N. has been caregiver to both her parents. She is a contributing writer to *Today's Caregiver Magazine.* She is the founder of the award-winning Web site "Kate's Place": http://home.att.net/~katesdrm/.

Carol Nahls is a parent and full-time, primary caregiver for her twenty-three-year-old daughter, who has severe brain injury.

Christine Nicholson, R.N., M.S.A., is presently the vice president of Product Development for Family Caring, Inc. d/b/a Boomerang. The company offers a work/life program for family caregiver support via an interactive Web site and call center. She has a background in nursing and geriatric care management. She has written and published articles on caregiving and related subjects for several years.

Michael T. Palermo, J.D., CFP has a private estate-planning practice and is a regular contributor to CBS Market Watch.com, as well as a seminar speaker on estate- and financial-planning issues. Mike maintains a popular and well-regarded Web site, "Crash Course in Wills & Trusts," www.mtpalermo.com.

Theresa R. Pantanella is the founder of Florida Aquatic Therapy and Exercise. She has specialized in aquatic rehabilitation for the past four years of her thirteen-year career in rehabilitation. Theresa has served as adjunct faculty for the Occupational Therapy Program at Barry University and is the certified trainer for the Broward County Arthritis Foundation in Aquatic Exercise.

Judd L. Parsons lives in Boynton Beach, Florida, with his wife Mindy, a breast cancer survivor, and their twins, Cody and Savannah. According to Mindy, Judd was her "rock" as she underwent three surgeries and six months of chemotherapy when their twins were just two years old.

The Reverend Steve Pieters has survived AIDS since 1982. He served for many years as a chaplain in hospitals and hospices, and as the director of AIDS Ministry for the Universal Fellowship of Metropolitan Community Churches. Pieters has published numerous articles on living with AIDS, as well as the autobiographical *I'm Still Dancing: A Gay Man's Health Experience.*

Michael Plontz is a staff writer for *Today's Caregiver Magazine.*

Brenda Race began writing poetry when she was caring for her mother, who had Alzheimer's disease. Her work examines both her feelings and what she feels her mother felt from the inside looking out. Her main goal is to help others who are caring for a loved one so that they may know there is hope and light at the end of a dark tunnel.

Vincent M. Riccardi, M.D., M.B.A., founder of American Medical Consumers (a patient advocate company), coaches and tutors medical consumers. He can be contacted at (818) 957-3508.

Jo Horne Schmidt is the author of *Caregiving: Helping an Aging Loved One,* hailed as "the book caregivers have been waiting for" when it was published in 1985. She has written three other books on aging and developed curriculum for university programs. Her husband pioneered adult day care in Wisconsin. Today, Jo continues to write and teach.

Nancy Schonwalter is managing editor of *Today's Caregiver Magazine*.

M. Ross Seligson, Ph.D., P.A. is a licensed psychologist in Ft. Lauderdale, Florida.

Senior Alternatives publishes free semiannual guides to senior housing around the nation. Contact them at (800) 350-0770 or www.senioralternatives.com.

Sandy Senor retired from the military and from a second career in banking. He has been caregiver to his wife, Nikki, who suffered a major stroke in August 1996. They live in Price, Utah, and enjoy traveling in their motor home.

Gary Slavin has been writing poetry as both an amateur and professional since his days in college. He has published articles on technical training, marketing, and sales for numerous business publications.

Dr. Gerald Trigg is the senior minister at First Methodist Church in Colorado Springs, Colorado.

Terry Weaver, M.P.S., N.H.A., C.M.C., A.C.C. has over twenty years of experience in health care, focusing on the needs of the older adult and caregiver. She is a certified care manager specializing in health care administration with a graduate degree in geriatric care management. Ms. Weaver founded GeriCare Associates in 1994 and can be reached at www.tlweaver@bellsouth.net.

Dorothy Womack, writer, poet, and author, was caregiver to her mother for fourteen years.

Katherine Dorn Zotovich is the mother of four and was caregiver for her parents for nearly a decade. As a caregiver, counselor, and literacy expert, she is the author of *Good Grief for Kids* and *My Memory Maker* journals. She is the creator of Journalkeepers.com, an Internet site that is geared to caregivers and their children.

The Fearless Caregiver Manifesto

I will fearlessly assess my personal strengths and weaknesses, work diligently to bolster my weaknesses, and graciously recognize my strengths.

I will fearlessly make my voice be heard with regard to my loved one's care, and be a strong ally to those professional caregivers committed to caring for my loved one and a fearless shield against those not committed to caring for my loved one.

I will fearlessly not sign or approve anything I do not understand, and will steadfastly request the information I need until I am satisfied with the explanations.

I will fearlessly ensure that all of the necessary documents are in place for my wishes and my loved one's wishes to be met in case of a medical emergency. These include durable medical powers of attorney, wills, trusts, and living wills.

I will fearlessly learn all I can about my loved one's health care needs and become an integral member of his or her medical care team.

I will fearlessly seek out other caregivers or care organizations and join an appropriate support group; I realize that there is strength in numbers and will not isolate myself from those who are also caring for their loved ones.

I will fearlessly care for my physical and emotional health as well as I care for my loved one's, I will recognize the signs of my own exhaustion and depression, and I will allow myself to take respite breaks and to care for myself on a regular basis.

I will fearlessly develop a personal support system of friends and family and remember that others also love my loved one and are willing to help if I let them know what they can do to support my caregiving.

I will fearlessly honor my loved one's wishes, as I know them to be, unless these wishes endanger his or her health or mine.

I will fearlessly acknowledge when providing appropriate care for my loved one becomes impossible because of either his or her condition or my own and seek other solutions for my loved one's caregiving needs.

— Gary Barg

Introduction

There are only four kinds of people in the world:
  Those who have been caregivers
  Those who are currently caregivers
  Those who will be caregivers
  Those who will need caregivers.

— Rosalynn Carter, *Helping Yourself Help Others*

In June 1990, three months after he retired, my father was diagnosed with bone marrow cancer. My mother went from wife and partner in a business venture they had just started to medic, nurse, mother, insurance and Medicare expert, and life support system for this proud and independent man. A year and a half later (shortly after my father passed away), her stepmother suffered a stroke and there was Mom, once again, caregiver-at-large. With me living in North Carolina at the time, a brother in New Orleans, and a sister with two small children to handle, my mother was virtually going it alone. We helped as much as we could, yet none of us could know the full scope of her day-to-day life as a caregiver.

By the time my grandfather started needing my mother's help as well, I was able to come back home to lend a hand. In doing the research necessary to help my own family, I kept running into people with the same look in their eyes as my mother had. All were searching for the right combination of answers that would make this loving labor just that much easier. But, as we were all to find out, the act of caregiving is not unlike trying to hang onto Jell-O®; it keeps shifting in your hands and there is just no way to get a firm grasp on it. There seem to be no right answers, just too many questions.

If you find yourself knowing the meaning of initials you never did before: AZT, ALF, SSI; if you feel as if you are the only one who can possibly understand the stress you're going through; if you find yourself answering to relatives and step-relatives who want no more to do with the situation than go over the books or offer advice from afar—please understand that you are not alone, there are many tireless and loving professionals and committed organizations dedicated to fighting the maladies that afflict your loved ones.

Today's Caregiver Magazine was founded on the principle that there are many caregivers—the true heroes of this era—who are willing to share the benefit of their experience, to be a supportive shoulder and an understanding heart. In this book, we've gathered together some of the best information, tips, and hopes of caregivers around the country who have written for our magazine—professional, family, and volunteer caregivers. Whether your loved one is living with cancer, heart disease, multiple sclerosis, Alzheimer's, AIDS, or any other disease, you will find much in common with the caregivers here. And it is our sincere wish that you will find not only answers, but also a level of comfort and support.

As a caregiver, you play many roles in our society. You may be "parenting" a parent, or caring for a child who needs care for the rest of his or her life, or you may be directly responsible for a formerly independent spouse, relative, or friend. In any case, it is possible that you will have the same responsibilities and stress as any parent caring for an infant child—possibly even changing diapers and bathing—for as long as you are a primary caregiver, no matter how old you are, no matter how old your loved one is.

With each new stage in your loved one's condition, your need for information is immediate and intense. But, more important, you need to learn how to use this new information, to interact successfully with health care professionals, insurance providers, other family members—and even with your loved one. You need to be well acquainted with all aspects of his or her care and make sure that your voice is heard by the health care system. You need to become fearless in caring for your loved one.

That is another aim of this book: to teach you to be a *fearless caregiver,* one who stands up to the system when the system no longer stands up for your loved one. Gone are the days when caregivers can simply rely on the family doctor to do the work of caring for their loved one; many of these decisions and costs are now the responsibility of the family. And in a way, this can be a good thing. It forces us to shift the established health care hierarchy, by necessity, to take a more active role in our loved one's care. But, this responsibility can come with a high price for caregivers. Too many caregivers die from a combination of stress, depression, and ill health. Or they become unable to care for themselves, let alone their loved ones, leaving a larger question of the health care system unanswered: Who will care for both caregiver and loved one, when the caregiver becomes ill?

It is my hope and intention that, after reading this book, you will have the skills and confidence to know if your loved one's care is appropriate, if the doctor treating your loved one is really the right doctor, if something more is needed. You will know not only how to ask for it, but also how to obtain services from the right people. You will know how to deal successfully with managed care organizations, home health services, and even your loved one. We even expect you will find yourself to be much more effective in enlisting the assistance you need from long distance caregivers and other members of the care team.

Caregivers can be heard in today's health care system. And we can be listened to. We have found significant common ground among the caregivers who are being heard. First, they believe that they can make a difference. Second, they see their role in their loved one's care as being just as important as any of the professional caregivers. And, third, they ask questions. They ask lots of questions. They research and do not easily take no for an answer. They have become *fearless caregivers.*

Fearless caregivers ask questions of their doctor and do not rest until they receive clear and concise answers. Fearless caregivers know their rights concerning their loved one's insurance plan and are able to exercise those rights. Fearless caregivers know how to find the latest treatment options and present qualified research to the members of their loved one's care team. Fearless caregivers are members of their loved one's care team. This book presents a lot of options, challenges, and opportunities to reestablish a more secure foothold on your corner of the world.

But, if you really don't believe you have the right to take these steps, it won't do you any good to read further. So we have to start here, at the beginning. We have to start with what we believe about ourselves, our rights, and our power. If you continue this journey with us, we can assure you that this will be the first step toward making the system work better for you and your loved one. This will be the first step in becoming an integral member of your loved one's care team: to becoming a fearless caregiver.

In 1994, I returned to Miami from Atlanta to help my mom as she cared for my grandparents. Since 1990, when my dad retired at sixty-one and was diagnosed almost immediately with bone marrow cancer, my mom had been the family's official caregiver. By 1994, my grandfather had been living with Alzheimer's disease for at least two years, and my grandmother had been in and out of the hospital battling the effects of a series of ministrokes.

It happened after a visit to my grandmother, during one of her frequent trips to the hospital. I was up to my elbows in brochures about adult living facilities, insurance information from the state, and product circulars from durable medical equipment companies. Suddenly it occurred to me that more could—and should—be done to make caregiving more comprehensible. Plumbers have magazines, bankers have magazines, why not caregivers? Why not? Mostly because the caregiver, with notable exceptions, had not been seen as anything but "the person pushing the wheelchair" by the health care system. For the most part, we were not seen as a constituency. We were not seen as a group of people with an intense need for information and support. We were not seen as we are: people in need of community.

We founded *Today's Caregiver Magazine* and www.caregiver. com to provide places for those with information and stories of value for caregivers to share their wisdom, not only for our potential readers but because we, as a family, desperately needed such wisdom ourselves. Over the past six years of publishing *Today's Caregiver Magazine* and hosting caregiver. com, one thing has become crystal clear: There is a path for caregivers to follow. While no two caregiving situations are the same—your loved one is not like anyone else, and your love and care for that person is unique—there are guidelines that, if followed, will make any caregiving situation easier to handle. We have chosen the best supportive information, articles, advice, and tips and techniques from the past six years of *Today's Caregiver Magazine* and asked our contributors to update their information. We have added new instructive commentary to bring you the most comprehensive guide to caring for your loved one.

In other words, we have put everything we can into *The Fearless Caregiver* to help you get rid of your own fears... to help you become a fearless caregiver. Is it easy? No. Is it something that can happen overnight? Wouldn't that be nice! Like anything else worthwhile, it will take work. Does the fear ever return? Yes, but you can learn how to fight it. Can this information help you to become a better caregiver to your loved one and yourself? I guarantee it.

The fear is yours to conquer. We will show you how.

— Gary Barg

Chapter 1

The Early Days

The Caregiver's Angel

Angels come in many forms,
and each one serves the Lord.
They teach us lessons of His love
and bring His Holy Word
From Heaven unto Earth they fly
and whisper in our ears
Songs of everlasting joy to last us through the years.
So when you hear the whistling wind
play music in the air,
remember there's an angel
singing songs for those who care.

— © Paul Dammann

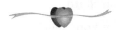

You Have the Right

There really is a secret to being the best caregiver you can possibly be: Learn from those caregivers who have gone before you. That's it. It's simple. Like most great truths it is almost too simple. No matter how unique your loved one's medical or emotional challenges are, millions of professional and family caregivers have walked in your shoes. Some of them have learned lessons of great value to you, and many of them are eager to share with those willing to listen.

These caregivers have trod the rocky path to a smoother road. They have had those sleepless nights, worrying about not asking the right questions of the doctor, worrying about not choosing the proper care facility for their loved ones, worrying about not being able to fight the system for appropriate care when necessary. They and many like them have spent their lives teaching caregivers how to best navigate the system, how to become fearless caregivers.

The Caregiver's Bill of Rights

Here is the first piece of wisdom—The Caregiver's Bill of Rights. Whether you are a new or experienced caregiver, you have the right to . . .

- Take care of yourself. This is not an act of selfishness. It will give you the capacity to take better care of your loved one.

- Seek help from others even though your loved one may object. You recognize the limits of your own endurance and strength.

- Maintain facets of your own life that do not include the person you care for, just as you would if he or she were healthy. You know that you do everything you reasonably can for this person, and you have the right to do some things just for yourself.

- Get angry, be depressed, and express other difficult feelings occasionally.

- Reject any attempts (either conscious or unconscious) by your loved one to manipulate you through guilt and/or depression.

- Receive consideration, affection, forgiveness, and acceptance for what you do for your loved one for as long as you offer these qualities in return.

- Take pride in what you are accomplishing and applaud the courage it has sometimes taken to meet the needs of your loved one.

- Protect your individuality and your right to make a life for yourself that will sustain you when your loved one no longer needs your full-time help.

- Expect and demand that as new strides are made in finding resources to aid physically and mentally impaired persons in our country, similar strides will be made toward aiding and supporting caregivers.

— © Jo Horne

This Bill of Rights, created in 1987 by Jo Horne, is just as valuable today as when it was first written. You need to consider this Bill of Rights as your Emancipation Proclamation. Freedom from guilt. Freedom from uncertainty. Freedom to care about yourself as well as your loved one.

Furthermore, as a caregiver, you have every right to have . . .

- Life made easier for you and your loved one.

- Your questions answered.

- Your opinions respected after you have made informed decisions.

- Your schedule considered.
- Your needs taken into account.

Once you understand these basic rights, you will understand your vital role in the caregiving process, and things will start falling into place.

Step One: Trust Your Instincts

You know more than you think you do; trust your instincts. And don't feel you have to be a hero. If the situation begins to put a strain on you, get help. Accept the help that people offer and suggest specific things that they can do for you. Ask one of them to sit with your loved one for a few hours. Ask another to pick up groceries. Tell Tom that, yes, you would love to have him cook dinner one night. Invite Mary to come over and just talk.

Establish a personal support system of friends and family. Hand out the responsibilities to each according to his or her abilities. If your sister is an accountant, ask her to handle the books. If your brother is an occupational therapist, ask him to work with your loved one on relearning an old living skill. If your cousin is a lawyer, ask her to help you review all the legal arrangements. Don't feel you have to do it all.

I know, I know, I can hear you saying, "What does he know? I'm the only one who knows how to care for Mom [or Dad or my sister or son]. Why should I bother with trying to get anyone else to help? Besides, my brother (the bum) would never lift a hand."

This mind-set was illustrated dramatically to me in a recent phone call. It was early evening when the phone rang in my office. As I began to lift the receiver to my ear, I could hear that the caller had already started a one-sided conversation.

"How dare he, I know everything I need to know about caring for my own mother."

"Hello?" I answered tentatively.

"I want you to give my brother his money back."

"Excuse me?"

"My brother had the nerve to send me a copy of *Today's Caregiver Magazine,* like he thought I needed anyone's help. I care for my mom and don't have time to read the paper. How do you think I'd have time to read a magazine?"

"I'll reimburse your brother, but please, let me offer you a free subscription. I would hope that in each issue there might be one thing which might help you."

"No! What can you tell me that I don't know? I know when to feed her, when to change her, and I don't have time for anyone who wants to help me."

Wow, what a statement: "I don't have time for anyone who wants to help me." Well, as a caregiver myself, I truly understood her feelings and frankly had thought those thoughts myself in the past. The funny thing is, once I understood that people really did want to help and I learned how to ask specific people for specific things, I was never turned down. That is the first step in becoming a *fearless caregiver*: Know how to ask whom for what and when.

Remember, caring for yourself is job one for any caregiver. If you wear yourself out, who will take care of both you and your loved one?

Step Two: Changing Your Perspective

The doctor has at least twelve years of training. The nurse has four, and the case manager at least two. They all have training, but your job begins in an instant: the moment the doctor reports your loved one's prognosis, or the moment you realize your loved one can no longer take care of himself or herself without assistance. It is then that the fearless caregiver starts learning (very) quickly how to think like a professional caregiver.

The diagram in Figure 1 represents the traditional paradigm in caregiving. The doctor acts as chief executive officer, or president, along with a secondary level of care professionals. Your loved one is below both levels of professional caregivers, and you (if you are lucky) are set off to the side, with a dotted line connecting you to your loved one. This paradigm does not make the best use of your talents and skills, and it is no longer valid.

The diagram in Figure 2 represents a more effective paradigm, one that makes your loved one the driving force of action and includes you as part of the care team. You are a dedicated member of this team, as important as the social worker, the therapist, and sometimes even the doctor. Each professional has his or her own job role and responsibilities, and yours is being a fearless caregiver for your loved one—a tireless and knowledgeable advocate and devoted giver of daily care.

You have become the most significant human being in the life of your loved one, and that gives you power. Along with that power comes responsibility. You now have to learn all you can about caring for your loved one. You have to stand up for your loved one, when necessary. If something seems wrong, unfair, awkward, inappropriate, or it's just not what you want or expect, you do have the right to do something about it. More important, it is your responsibility to do something about it.

Once you actually believe this, speaking up will become easier. Getting people to do things they should have done in the first place will become second nature. When you understand that you deserve the best people have to offer, you will function within that belief. And, miraculously, as people understand that you truly subscribe to this paradigm, they

Figure 1. **Traditional Caregiver Paradigm**

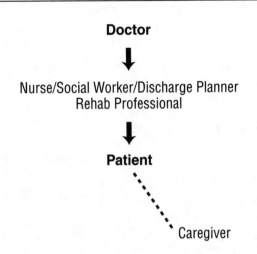

Figure 2. **Fearless Caregiver Paradigm**

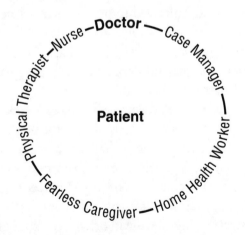

begin to fall in line with your expectations. But, this cannot be lip service on your part; you really have to believe in your right and your power.

If you don't believe that you and your loved one deserve the best the system has to offer, why should anyone else think you deserve it?

Reframing Your Perspective

You know your rights as a caregiver, and you are beginning to understand where you really belong in the care team. You have a concept, at this point, of your responsibility to your loved one, and you have a better picture of the care team's responsibility to you. You are in uniform, you have your supplies. Now we start training.

The next step in becoming your loved one's fearless caregiver is what we call *reframing perspective*. You must change your perspective from that of an interested and loving observer, to a fully empowered fearless caregiver, the one who makes sure that everything that can be done for your loved one is done. You need to believe that the new fearless caregiver paradigm is possible.

Frightened by your new role? Repeat after me: I will probably experience stress and depression as a caregiver. This is normal and perfectly acceptable.

What should not be acceptable, however, is to let the stress and depression control you. According to the National Family Caregivers Association, more than 63 percent of all caregivers say that stress is their most common feeling. Our goal is for you to become one of the 37 percent who do not fall into that group, so you can put your head down on your pillow every night knowing that even though life as a caregiver can still be difficult and heartbreaking, you have done everything possible to help your loved one for one more day. And, sometimes, frankly, that's good enough.

— Gary Barg

Suddenly

It has been written that "all men are created equal," but it never said for just how long. One day we are all equal, and the next day one of us is not. One day we are laughing, loving, playing together—and overnight we are not.

You both go to sleep, happily looking forward to a bright tomorrow, only to find that tomorrow has changed from a bright-looking future to feeling as if you have smashed into a solid brick wall. Suddenly one of you may not have any future. Where do you go, what do you do, how do you do it, can you afford to do it? Horrible, horrible decisions fall into your lap—and all of this happens virtually overnight.

I can tell you from my own experience: after the initial shock of the diagnosis, fear—downright, nerve-racking fear—creeps into your soul. Then you realize that your world, and your loved one's, has tumbled upside down, like a carnival ride. But no one's laughing.

As a caregiver for one you love, you want to do everything as well as humanly possible. In many instances, you are alone; the people outside of your immediate family do not want to be involved in the hardships of being a caregiver. All some of these people want to know is how the money is being spent. Don't count on them for any moral, physical, or financial help, just lip service, which they give freely.

Caregiver—the word says exactly what it means. Your life is devoted to taking care of another life. Suddenly, it seems as if everything is happening at once, but try to take one step at a time. Take time to give care to the caregiver. If you don't, the carefully constructed house of cards you are building can tumble down around your ears, and you can't afford that luxury because you are desperately needed by your charge and the rest of your family.

Take a moment to consider what would happen if you were not there to do your caregiving, how your situation would look from the outside in. You are indispensable. Keep yourself as physically, mentally, and spiritually fit as possible; otherwise you'll have to find a caregiver for yourself. I know this as a past, present, and future caregiver.

— Monica Weiss Barg

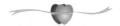

Levels of Adjustment

When a family member faces a chronic illness, the entire family structure is rocked to its foundation. The inevitable life changes occur in stages, and we can adjust to them more easily if we recognize these stages when they happen. Having experienced the trauma of my husband's paralysis following surgery, I have learned to identify three major levels of adjustment. It is important to acknowledge these and understand that we have choices at each of these levels.

The first level of adjustment is accepting the responsibility for our family member through the initial medical crisis, release from the hospital, and beyond. The momentary pleasure of having him or her home is soon replaced with abject fear of the enormous job ahead. No instruction manual is sent home, and even the simplest tasks take on Herculean proportions. The types of choices to be made include personal care needs, everyday household management, a plan for disease management, and the level of physical activity permitted. Fortunately, help is available through home health agencies and community programs.

The second level is the reorganization of the home—physically, financially, and in the roles family members play. When our loved one arrives home, it may be necessary to acquire home medical equipment such as a hospital bed and make alterations to accommodate a wheelchair, lift, or walker. If our loved one has been the main breadwinner, the family's financial support will suddenly fall to someone else. Major role changes are called for. Both the care recipient and caregiver will feel insecure at first with the loss of the old roles and uncomfortable with their new roles, until they become more familiar.

The third level is the most difficult level of adjustment. Caregiver, care recipient, and other family members must accept the changes this new situation demands. In time, this regime becomes normal. But at first, everyone is in shock with the realization that their circumstances are permanent. Acceptance will come with time, if the family works together.

The entire family must take a proactive role in seeking out educational and support resources and accepting the family's reconfiguration. This journey will be easier and more productive when everyone concentrates on where you are going, rather than on where you have been.

— Juli A. Koroly

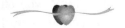

What Does a Caregiver Need to Know?

It starts with changes. At first, it's just little things. Like having to mow the lawn, going to the grocery, having to be transportation for a trip to the doctor—a funny feeling when you're on the phone that maybe something isn't right.

Maybe subtle differences—your wife doesn't seem to have the energy to do things the way she used to—the kitchen's not clean and the laundry's not done.

Then worry—variations in behavior or medical circumstances—your husband just isn't the same or your wife isn't taking care of herself the way she always did.

But, no one seems concerned yet—except you!

Then it happens—the stroke was so sudden, no warning—what will happen? What does the doctor mean?

Now you're a caregiver—welcome to family caregiving!

Caregivers Need to Know

When we step in to provide help to family or friends, we don't think of it as "caregiving." We're just helping out, doing what people do for each other. But when individuals no longer are sure how to help each other or the helping becomes frustrating, confusing, or too time or physically consuming—then our role changes and we become caregivers.

Recent studies indicate that one in every four families is providing care to an elder or other loved one. This care may be in the form of financial help; homemaking or household repairs; transportation; or actual, hands-on personal care.

When we become involved in caregiving, depending on the caregiving situation and involvement, the flavor of relationships, the nature of activities and everyday routines begin to change. Perhaps that involvement is providing direct care such as housekeeping or assistance with bathing. Perhaps it's providing long distance emotional support—frequent phone calls, cards, and visits. Or, perhaps others are in control and ignore your concerns and you can only stand aside and worry.

Be aware that caregiving for another is a part of life today. Further, there are resources to aid the special needs that caregivers have and support the decisions they have to make.

> The family caregiver is responsible for and impacted by the practical, physical, emotional, financial, social, and medical needs and limitations of a chronically ill, disabled, elderly or frail family member or other loved one.
>
> — David Levy, President, Family Caring, Inc.

When You're a Caregiver

Caregiving takes on many faces. Each situation is unique. One may be caring for a parent, a spouse, or an adult child with disabilities. A caregiver may be an only child or perhaps have physical or mental limitations of his or her own—yet have full responsibility for the care of another. The care receiver may be close by or live thousands of miles away.

Many of us will first enter caregiving in a time of crisis. For others, there is ample warning of the coming need for help—perhaps due to a chronic condition or severe injury. As the caregiving role is assumed, the caregiver will be asked to respond to many new activities and circumstances. In order to meet the challenge on a continuing basis:

- Caregivers need to know what the problems are and what can be expected.

- Caregivers need to know what can realistically be done about the problems they face.

- Caregivers need to know how to find the best information and services.

- Caregivers need to know how to find advice that can be trusted.

We all face change in our own way. Sometimes elders will cling to old ideas and issues of independence in what seem to be foolish or unsafe ways. Anger and denial are often present when things must change, affecting feelings and actions in unexpected ways.

Individuals diagnosed with chronic illness find their own way to manage. Many times it is done by collecting information and strength from those around them and from past experiences. Sometimes, the response is heroic—sometimes, the choice is an unhealthy one. Most often, people and families work hard to make the best of an illness or disability by making accommodations and providing encouragement. Essentially, living life to the fullest as much as possible is surely the goal. Caregivers and care receivers have a special relationship to one another. Remember that each in his or her own way is a giver and a receiver of attention, kindness, and love.

Caregivers need to develop a comprehensive care recipient support network to aid in keeping life as planned, organized, and efficient as possible. In order to know what one is faced with, information must be gathered from many sources. Physicians, nurses, social workers, and other therapists may be available to give assistance. Federal agencies and national disease organizations are excellent sources of practical advice and may provide support groups or other networking opportunities. One's personal caregiving network should include not only the loved one's health care providers, but the vendors of goods and services that are needed to maintain his or her daily routine. It is just as important for the caregiver to add to the support network the people or groups that he or she can turn to for caregiver help and support.

If one is a long distance caregiver, knowing the names and telephone numbers of a loved one's neighbors, friends, and faith community is also important. Communication, however, is a two-way street—caregivers need to be easily reached by the many people who are involved in the support and care of a loved one.

Planning is important and caregivers can begin by locating community services, organizations, and local agencies that may be needed in the future. Caregivers also need to become familiar with insurance plans, legal and financial documents, assistive devices, and other products designed to help frail elders or those with disabilities to function at their highest level.

Since chronic illness or disabling conditions are, by their nature, long lasting, caregiving situations are ever changing. A treatment, therapy, or service that was right for yesterday is not necessarily going to be right for tomorrow. Even within a stable period, various options should be investigated that might improve upon the current situation.

These options may include home care, companion service, senior centers, and alternative therapies such as chiropractic, acupuncture, or massage. Repairs or modifications may increase the safety of the home environment, enabling an individual to remain in his or her home rather than have to seek an institutional type of living facility.

It is often difficult to think of new ways to do things, particularly when one is under stress. We all have a tendency to keep things the way they are during those times. However, finding other ways of "caring" may be of benefit to both caregiver and care receiver. Many alternatives can potentially increase the quality of life for a loved one by providing interesting activities and increasing physical or mental well-being, thereby increasing the independence and quality of life for all involved.

An essential skill to be developed is learning to *take care of the caregiver.* Too many caregivers expect that they can "do it all"—an attitude that may lead to burnout and unnecessary health-related problems. It is important to spend some time each day in both physical and spiritual/emotional activities to reduce stress, think clearly, and maintain a generous spirit.

It is important to learn as much as possible about a loved one's condition and the medical/social plans for treatment:

- What can be expected in the future?

- What are the warning signs of problems?

- What are the best ways to provide assistance and encouragement?

- Have there been changes to the financial capability of the family?

- Is there the time, energy, or skills to provide the assistance needed?

- Will there be changes in work schedules or to other commitments?

- What will happen to other relationships?

Developing a realistic approach takes time, knowledge, commitment, and good communication between all parties. Knowing what to expect allows us to think about how to cope—to be prepared. This approach helps to manage expectations. It helps avoid providing too much or too little assistance in the present and helps both caregiver and care receiver to plan for future needs and activities. For caregivers and their families, as well as the care receiver, this is a long-term process—sometimes painful, sometimes exhausting, often a most rewarding time of family life.

Talking to each other about one's wishes for future care and what plans have already been implemented should be a high priority for each family before a crisis occurs. Caregiving has become another phase of life, like getting married or having children—it's essential to be prepared.

— Christine Nicholson, R.N., M.S.A.

Maintaining Emotional Intimacy When Your Loved One Is Ill

In our culture, when we discuss intimacy, many people think immediately of sexuality. While sex may be part of an intimate relationship, it in no way encompasses it. When we think of intimacy as only sex, it makes it difficult to focus on the other really satisfying parts of human relationships.

Development of truly intimate relationships is difficult during times of good health and well-being. When someone is chronically or terminally ill, and is being provided physical care, that person can find it very difficult to ask to have his or her emotional needs met as well. Caregivers are often overwhelmed and may have difficulty verbalizing their own emotional and physical needs. There may be feelings of guilt and shame attached to having any physical or emotional needs.

The primary concern of caregivers remains how to keep their relationship with their loved one at a level that enables emotional intimacy. In counseling sessions we advise our clients to remember the three As:

Acknowledgment

Good communication is the key to acknowledging your loved one. Remember, to communicate effectively you need to accept your differences, listen to each other's opinions, and not close the door on painful subjects, including the wants and desires of the caregiver.

If your loved one is terminally ill, he or she may want to discuss feelings about death. We would encourage you, as the caregiver, to be prepared for the inevitable and invite discussion whenever possible. As the caregiver, acknowledge the person's feelings and be supportive of his or her view of the situation. Be careful not to take the attitude, "I know what is best" or "Do what I say."

Attention

Paying attention to someone involves a lot more than monitoring his or her physical well-being. You can let a person know that you are paying attention by listening attentively, making good eye contact, and being aware of nonverbal communication, including body position, tension, and lack of eye contact.

Affection

Emotional intimacy can be maintained through the simplest of physical gestures: a kiss on the cheek or forehead, coupled with a warm smile, a back rub, brushing the patient's hair, or just saying, "I love you."

In an intimate relationship, both parties have to maintain a balance between closeness and separateness. This allows people to maintain their individuality *and* a sense of intimacy. The caregiver and patient can sustain a quality of intimacy similar to what they had before the illness. Having a healthy respect for the other's situation is crucial to all relationships.

As the caregiver, you have emotional needs that your loved one cannot always meet because of his or her condition. You need to recognize that having your own needs does not take away from the wonderful relationship you had or may still have with your loved one. They are a sign of your own humanness. Caregivers need to maintain a network of outside support by keeping relationships with family members and friends who can provide them with the acknowledgment, attention, and affection caregivers need and deserve. Taking care of these emotional needs will allow you to focus on your loved one with a relaxed, positive, loving attitude.

— Louise Center, L.C.S.W. and Jennifer Kay, L.C.S.W.

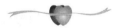

Long Distance Caregiver— Coping with Emotions

Being a long distance caregiver presents a unique set of problems. The emotional drain of being too far from a loved one to be of direct help can be devastating. How can one describe the fear that envelops you when the phone rings and the call tells of yet another crisis with your loved one? It is something you learn to live with every day. However, you are never ready for that call. I understand because I have been both a long distance and now a full-time primary caregiver. We all feel the same emotions: guilt, anger, frustration, and isolation. They just differ as our individual caregiver roles differ.

As a long distance caregiver, I had to struggle with my guilt over not being there all the time, or not being able to ensure that proper care was provided on a regular basis. While I learned to deal with these issues, I think I was never really comfortable with them. Many times I felt isolated because I would learn of a change after the fact, and usually after I could have been of help. That leads to a feeling of being fragmented from the family. Eventually, it is easy to see how such a family member might not offer any advice or help at all. Or if a family member does offer it, often it is not very practical in the eyes of the primary caregiver because the person could have no idea of what the loved one wants or needs. In time this fragmentation can and often does lead to anger with siblings, which is the last thing that should happen. This is a time when families need to grow closer and share the good and the bad.

Now, as primary caregiver, I have had to face just that issue. I have had to look at my siblings and understand that while they can't be here, it does not diminish the concern they may feel for our father. From this perspective, I would like to mention a few things that all family members can do to help ensure that proper care is provided to their loved one. As long distance caregiver, you have an opportunity to offer a much-needed respite to your sibling. It may be difficult, but arrange for regular visits so that the primary caregiver has a break. A week or two several times a year is a wonderful gift to your sibling and allows you to be an active member of the care team.

The primary caregiver has an obligation as well. You need to keep lines of communication open with those family members who don't live locally. Offer regular updates on your loved one's condition and include the other members as much as possible in the decision-making process. Remembering that you do not have to carry the whole load and letting other family members know that you need their input is essential. And it will go a long way toward lessening the fear of a telephone call late at night.

— Catherine Murphy, R.N.

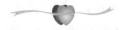

Caregivers and the Internet

Five years ago, when I first typed the word *caregiver* into a search engine, I was shocked to find so few results. There were fewer than a hundred listings and none related to emotional support for the caregiver. Most of the listed sites contained very good information about caring for the elderly and their related diseases. The sites talked about things like stress and caregiver burnout, yet did not offer any practical solutions to the caregiver.

Try typing that same word into a search engine today and see what happens. I did recently, and one search engine alone produced thousands of Web pages from which to choose!

Quite a difference in a few short years, wouldn't you say? It speaks volumes about how far we have come as caregivers. Literally thousands of us have been empowered through the Internet. Caregivers seek out the answers to the difficult questions regarding health care alternatives, legal issues, and trying to find a connection with others in similar situations to get emotional and spiritual support. More important, they have discovered a way to find some refuge and bond with other caregivers.

You can see this on each Web site you visit. Look at the number of visitors to the site. Many number in the thousands and in some cases, hundreds of thousands. The love and warmth that one experiences is inspirational to many who visit.

I have talked to Webmasters about these sites and why they were created. Consistent throughout was a strong desire to help and support other caregivers. In addition, many of these same Webmasters felt compelled to build the site out of their own need for support. Like me, they realized that if we feel these emotions and concerns, there had to be many other caregivers out there who were having the same trouble finding support and encouragement.

While many caregivers were able to find help with some of the more practical issues of caregiving, they still felt a need for emotional support. It is not easy for others who are not in similar situations to understand the nature of the emotional stress that the caregiver deals with each day. The longer you are in the role, the more important it becomes to find outlets for your bottled-up feelings. Without these outlets, the door is left open to caregiver burnout, and medical problems frequently result.

Until a few years ago, finding this support for many was literally impossible. I know because I was one of the masses who spent sleepless nights wondering why being a caregiver was so difficult, or why no one seemed to understand what I was going through on a personal level. There were times when I felt I could not go on, and then felt guilty for thinking I wanted out of this role I voluntarily accepted.

I can still remember the night when, in desperation, I sat down at my computer and typed in the word *caregiver.* As I browsed through the listed sites, I found information about many issues. However, none of it seemed to help resolve the pain I was feeling. It occurred to me that if I could be feeling this way, there had to be others who shared the same need.

One of the first sites I found was a caregiver bulletin board. This was a place where one could post questions or comments and have an opportunity to reply to postings already on the board. I found myself posting a comment that night. I introduced myself as a caregiver in search of support and invited other caregivers to visit my first feeble attempt at a Web page. The rest, as they say, "is history." I began to hear from other caregivers in a variety of situations. All were seeking the same thing. They were searching for someone who could understand what they were going through, and a friend they could talk to openly and honestly about these feelings. Many of the caregivers I met then are still a large part of my life, and while our roles have changed in multiple ways, the love and support we shared goes on.

Today more and more caregivers are turning to the Internet as a source of support and education. There are Web sites that provide informational and interactive arenas for the caregiver. As a matter of fact, there are whole caregiver communities being developed on the Internet that were not there just a few short years ago. In addition, there are sites that tell the caregivers' own stories, often in the form of a journal. However you wish to categorize these sites, they all have one common thread: They were created out of a desire to help others cope with the everyday issues of caregiving.

Despite this, there are those who feel the Internet plays a small role in helping the caregiver. After all, not every caregiver has the means to afford a computer or time to spend on it. As a result, many continue to have little or no support. If it were in my power, I would supply every caregiver with a computer, because I believe the Internet is a powerful source of support and education. A man once told me that if it were not for the computer, he didn't think his wife would have survived the stress of caring for her mother at home. Throughout her mother's last painful days, his wife was able to share her experiences with others who knew what she was going through. She was able to talk about things that would have gone unsaid otherwise. And when her mother died, the support did not. The friends she had made on the Internet were there for her and still are. She went on to create her own Web page and continues to provide support to other caregivers online.

How did the Internet become popular to the caregiver? It became a refuge when caregivers found themselves unable to leave their homes to go to local support groups, if any existed in their area. They often had to work full-time jobs and provide care to their loved one. In many cases, there was little or no help to be found. Finding time to get to the store for groceries was a major problem, let alone trying to find someone to stay with their loved one so they could do something for themselves. They began to look to the Internet for answers to some of their questions.

What they also found was that they were not alone in what they were experiencing. Suddenly, the emotional roller coaster they were on seemed less scary. They discovered that there were others who felt as they did. They learned that anger, frustration, guilt, and depression are common to caregivers. And, more important, they discovered that other caregivers also tried to hide these emotions, because they felt it was wrong to have them. When given the chance to meet others in similar situations, and to learn that these feelings are normal, it was as though an enormous weight had been lifted from their shoulders. They found that it was okay to be angry. They learned ways to deal with the anger and even to turn it into joy and laughter. For many, the few minutes they were able to spend online each day became their primary source of contact with the outside world. And often this contact was late in the evening, once they had their loved one settled for the night.

In chat sessions—a major source of support for caregivers—it is not unusual to have to leave quickly to answer a call from a loved one. No one is censured for the disruption, and when the caregiver returns to the screen, more than likely a few extra minutes are spent making sure all is well with both caregiver and care recipient. In addition, the caregiver does not have to worry about finding someone to stay with the loved one so he or she can attend a support meeting. Caregivers meet online with other caregivers when it is convenient to them. Many of the online chat rooms today are open twenty-four hours a day. There is always somewhere one can find support when it is needed most.

On a personal level, the Internet saved my sanity. At a time in my life when I was on the edge and had no clue about how to pull back, the Internet gave me hope to continue. It brought me in contact with others who were also in desperate need of an understanding ear. I was able to move forward and become one of the countless caregivers devoted to increasing awareness to the needs of caregivers everywhere.

To the noncaregiver, this may seem like a strong statement. It is still difficult for one who has not walked in our shoes to fully comprehend the emotions and feelings surrounding the role of caregiver, even after all the public education in recent years on our needs. Nor is it easy to understand how valuable the Internet can be to the caregiver. In my case, I had no local support group to seek out, and there were no resources to fall back on for relief or respite. I could not leave my house whenever I wanted because there was no one to stay with Dad. And late at night when I could not sleep, the Internet was my refuge. It became the light at the end of my tunnel and, in return, I used what I had taught myself to try to help other caregivers.

In closing, I encourage each of you to look to the Internet as a source of support and learning. I am sure that when you do you will see how beneficial it can be. While the Internet can never replace the benefit of support in the "real world," isn't it nice to know it is there if you ever need it?

— Catherine Murphy, R.N.

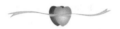

Finding the Faith to Meet the Challenge

Caring for an ailing loved one is an expression of love. It is a difficult task, however, and often unpleasant and stressful. Watching someone with whom we shared our lives waste away arouses a collision of feelings: compassion, pity, anxiety, frustration, resentment, and anger. People around us admire, even look up to us. But sometimes it becomes difficult to share our inner conflicts, our struggle with darker feelings and thoughts. We even start to become angry with ourselves for feeling the way we do; guilt interrupts our efforts. Our sadness is tinged by resentment; we are left with anguish. Because the efforts and energy involved in caring for a terminally or chronically ill family member are so great, we deplete ourselves. We sense that a part of ourselves has become infected by the dying process. We, too, begin to slip away from life.

Although we are all aware of support, just talking about our feelings appears to be insufficient. After a little bit of ventilation, the anguish returns. Neighbors or friends do not enter that bedroom with us each morning and throughout each day and night. They do not inhale the odor of imminent death. We discover that we live in a different world that has become a kind of parallel reality. Friends and neighbors still dine out and visit, attend concerts and movies. We, on the other hand, visit doctors and hospitals. We become relatively expert at medications and their side effects.

What sense of God we may have had at other times in our lives is radically diminished. We cannot communicate our faith because we are confused about what to pray for. We always believed that being good had its rewards. Misery was for bad people. We may begin to wonder if God is cruel, indifferent, or merely a childish illusion. Bad things do happen to good people, and, to add to our frustration, good things happen to bad people. I may lift up my eyes, to paraphrase the psalmist, but whence cometh my help?

I believe that faith and spirituality are very important in the lives of caregivers. Support groups allow us some time to ventilate, but beyond the slight release of psychic tensions we are desperately in need of meaning. What is the purpose of pain? What is the value of my caring? How can I find grace in all this misery? These are more than philosophical questions; they are essential for our very existence.

Ultimately, what enables us to live with our portion in life is our capacity for making it meaningful. This, of course, is the task of religion: to provide the structure or paradigm through which we discover meaning in our lives. The Talmud teaches: One must bless God for the bad in life as well as for the good. In the act of blessing God, we begin the deeply personal journey from senseless pain to meaningful challenge.

— Rabbi Saul Goldman

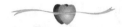

Chapter 2

Legal and Financial Matters

Déjà Vu

I stood in the hospital emergency room with my mother, the ER doctor, and the social worker. My mother and I had brought my ninety-one-year-old grandfather in just a few hours earlier. The next few words spoken by the social worker immediately jerked me back seven years to the night my father passed away. The same hospital, the same little group, and my mom and me with two health care professionals and the very same question, "Does he have a living will?"

I know the implication of these words was not lost on my mother either. My dad was literally on his deathbed, having battled multiple myeloma for a year and a half. He made his wishes about his end of life decision known, but we could never actually face seeing them on paper. Somehow, those papers were never signed.

I had slipped a copy of the living will into my back pocket, however, finally realizing that perhaps we would need to face the inevitable only hours before his passing.

My mother came to a similar realization. She asked me if I knew where we could find a copy of his living will. I'll never forget the expression on her face when I produced the papers on the spot. I still don't know if it was surprise or horror: perhaps a combination of the two. She signed with my father's power of attorney, and, perhaps realizing that the last piece was in place for his departure, my father passed away within the hour.

So, you would think that seven years later, we, of all people, would be prepared to answer that same question. After having created a magazine for caregivers, after convincing people through national television and radio shows across the nation to have living wills in place for themselves and their loved ones, after being caregivers for my grandparents for the past four years, you'd think we would be prepared. You would think that we would have microfiche copies of my grandfather's living will in each of our wallets. You'd think that the papers would have been signed years ago, since, not unlike my father, my grandfather had also let his wishes regarding his end of life be known.

The truth is, we looked at each other as if the past seven-year gap in time were mere minutes, and we suffered the same agony we had suffered all those years ago. Thankfully, we didn't need the papers—my grandfather recuperated from that event.

If I can wish anything beyond health and happiness for you and your loved ones, it is that you take the time to have your loved one's living will, health care surrogate, and DNR (do not resuscitate) wishes legally represented. And for the sake of your loved ones, fill out these forms for yourself, as well. Then, hopefully, all of your déjà vu's will be sweet ones.

— Gary Barg

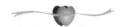

Top Ten Things for Caregivers to Start Doing Now

1. Keep records of all medications and reactions: make notes about what works, what doesn't, and when you informed the physician of any problems.

2. Keep records of all doctor appointments: the reason for the visit, the doctor's responses to our concerns, any procedures performed, etc.

3. Start or continue to maintain copies of medical records for your loved one, and for yourself. These will be beneficial should a grievance arise, or if there are questions about medical histories.

4. Plan for the unexpected: discuss the plans and wishes of everyone involved in the caregiving family. Talk about final resting places and what arrangements your family wants.

5. Have advance directives filled out and given to the primary physician and all relatives who may need the form.

6. Have a last will and testament completed or updated: without a signed will, the courts will decide how to distribute the possessions of your loved ones.

7. Keep a record of where all-important documents are kept. When an emergency or tragedy occurs, locating information should not be how we spend our thoughts and energies.

8. Record all financial information: investments, resources, creditors, debtors, business transactions, etc.

9. Have an insurance analysis done: Are your home, life, and health insurance still appropriate to your family's

needs? What about the insurance policies for your loved ones? Do you all have enough coverage to take care of any eventuality? Do you have provisions for long-term care? For respite care? Is your house adequately covered?

10. Clean out the medicine chest. Look for expiration dates on all medicine, and check with your doctor about medications prescribed earlier that will be harmful with current prescriptions or are no longer effective for you or your loved one. Not only will you save space, you might also save a life.

— Today's Caregiver Magazine

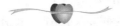

The Other Side of the Bed

In living with a person who is coping with a chronic illness, the needs of the patient and the needs of the caregiver are not always in harmony. The caregiver is looking for some respite and help with the chores of caregiving. The loved one may be seeking to maintain privacy, autonomy, and independence. Sometimes, this makes the patient seem selfish—not recognizing the time and effort devoted to her or him. Under normal circumstances, this extreme self-absorption is selfish, but not for a loved one with a long-term illness.

I discovered how intense the caregiver-patient conflict can be recently when I met with an ailing seventy-six-year-old man and his wife to talk about activating their home health insurance policy. The man was so weak that he had been having frequent falls and bleeding. For a year or so he had been in and out of the emergency room and hospital with serious medical conditions. His wife was exhausted.

Intellectually, he understood that it would be helpful for his wife to have someone come and do the extra laundry and pick up prescriptions, but he could not even fathom having that person in the house with him "just in case" while his wife did simple errands, although he knew that she was afraid to leave him alone because he often fell asleep in his chair and tumbled out of it.

"I have lived all my life independently," he insisted. "This is the way I want to continue living. I don't want people talking about me—saying that I don't understand what is happening or what I am talking about. And I don't like it when the nurses and doctors tell my wife what is going on and don't tell me."

I thought that was clear and well put. This problem is not an easy one to solve. I guess we all have to know what our bottom line is. I know a couple where the husband is in his forties and has Huntington's disease. The wife had a difficult time getting him to stop driving. Finally, she said, "You can drive or be married to me. It is your choice." He made a good decision and gave up driving.

One way to ensure that the wishes of the patient are respected and the onus of major decisions is taken off the caregiver's shoulders is to make a living will. The purpose of a living will is to address the needs, concerns, and wishes of the chronically ill person while he or she is able to make decisions, not only about death, but also how to be treated while still alive.

A living will answers such questions as:

1. Who would you like your health care surrogate to be?

2. What kinds of treatment would you like or not like?

3. How comfortable would you like to be made, and what would that look like for you?

4. How would you like others to treat you?

5. What would you want your loved ones to know when you are no longer able to tell them?

While these are admittedly hard discussions to have, they allow us to stay in tune with the person we are caring for. It allows that person to remain a person, rather than just a patient. I highly recommend that all families, even those not dealing with a chronic or life-threatening illness, take a look at a model living will called "Five Wishes." Currently thirty-three states recognize a Five Wishes will. I hope you and your family will consider using this important tool to help you begin a dialogue on these important matters. You can receive a model Five Wishes will by writing to:

> Aging with Dignity
> P.O. Box 1661
> Tallahassee, FL 32302-1661

> — Jennifer Kay, L.C.S.W.

Elements of the Estate Plan

Durable Power of Attorney (POA)

Coupled with a will and an advance medical directive (discussed later), the durable power of attorney (POA) is, for many people, a superior alternative to the simple living trust in planning for disability or incompetence. These documents are more familiar to folks than the concept of a trust, and their total cost is less than that of a trust.

Let us begin with a few general points. A POA is a document in which one person, the *principal,* gives authority to his or her *attorney in fact* (who need not be a lawyer) to act on his or her behalf. The scope of the power can be quite limited—for example, the purchase of a single real estate investment—or almost unlimited. The principal can even grant the power to make gifts of his or her property, but not to make a will. Note that *all* powers of attorney—even the "durable" variety described below—end at the death of the principal.

POAs can allow one to delegate broad authority over personal financial affairs, *except in the case of disability or incompetence.* For this, a *durable POA* is necessary. It is a very broad and detailed document that also states: "This POA shall not be affected by my subsequent disability or incapacity, or by the passage of time." This sentence is what makes it "durable"—even if the principal "takes a licking," this POA "keeps on ticking." Without that sentence, state law would probably render the POA inoperative immediately upon the disability of the principal—precisely when it is most needed.

You should understand that this kind of durable POA takes effect immediately. It does not wait until disability. Therefore, it is possible, in theory, for the attorney-in-fact to act independently, behind the principal's back, even if the principal is healthy. Some people find this thought unsettling, but it usually ought not to be. Presumably, of course, your attorney-in-fact is trustworthy beyond reproach. If there is any doubt about this, perhaps the durable POA is just not for you.

An alternative to this kind of durable POA is the *springing POA.* This is a type of durable POA that works, and is worded, differently. It *does* wait until disability, and only then "springs" into action. This can pose a big problem: There must be a formal determination of disability before the POA is considered operative and is accepted. At best, this means at least a short delay and expense. (A springing POA might provide, for example, that two doctors examine the principal and attest to his or her disability.) At worst, there might be uncertainty, disagreement, or squabbling among doctors and/or family over the degree of the principal's disability. Banks or others might balk at recognizing the authority of the attorney-in-fact for this reason. When this situation unfolds, the matter often winds up in court, which is the very thing you want to avoid.

The springing POA apparently is used because some people just feel uncomfortable making a delegation of power while they are still healthy. This is quite understandable, but the potential problems should be considered.

For a POA to be valid, the principal must be of sound mind when signing it, even if it is to remain valid during subsequent disability (that is, durable). The rules for determining adequate soundness of mind for a POA are probably not as clear-cut as for establishing testamentary capacity to make a will. State law might require *greater* mental capacity to prepare a valid POA than a will. Even so, a POA should be valid if signed during a lucid interval during a prolonged period of incompetence.

Guardianship

An unfortunate fact of life for the elderly is the possibility of mental and/or physical incapacity. *Guardianship* involves a proceeding in court and can be the less desirable alternative to *advance* planning for disability with a durable POA or living trust.

TIP: Although blank POA forms are readily available, this is a document best prepared by an attorney. The trouble with any POA is that it is presented to banks and other third parties who can arbitrarily decline to recognize it for their own reasons. It is important to recognize that the party being asked to accept your POA is doing you a favor. If he, she, or it has any reason whatsoever to fear "getting in trouble" for honoring the document, the POA might be rejected. A stock brokerage, for example, does not want to worry about following the instructions of an attorney-in-fact under a customer's POA only to have the customer file a lawsuit later, arguing that the document should not have been honored.

The relationship of the guardian to the person in his or her care (the ward) is much like that of parent to child. The law, quite rightly, considers it a very big deal to strip an adult of independence and impose that relationship on him or her.

For this reason, the process of obtaining court appointment as a guardian involves some time and money. Details vary by state, but there is probably an office in the local county court that handles guardianship. The first step is a "petition" to the court by someone asking to be appointed guardian. In some areas, the court clerk's office has blank forms and instructions so that people need not hire an attorney; usually, however, you will need one.

What happens next accounts for the unavoidable delay and, perhaps, expense. Although most people act with the best of motives, the court must make a serious inquiry into the *necessity* of full guardianship, or of guardianship limited to either the ward's person or property, as appropriate. Sometimes, for example, life would be more "convenient" for an adult child caregiver if he or she were the parent's legal guardian. That would not suffice, however, if the child sought guardianship and the parent objected.

The court generally requires a hearing, at which some kind of evaluation of the disabled person by medical and/or mental health professionals is presented. Often, the petitioner seeking guardianship must make arrangements and pay for the examination(s) and reports. Additionally, in most places, a lawyer is appointed by the court to represent the disabled person. This is a further safeguard to ensure that no competent person is "railroaded" just because he or she is too weak or intimidated to speak out.

Living Wills and Other Advance Medical Directives (AMDs)

These documents address a variety of complicated medical, legal, and ethical situations that may confront each of us near the end of life. Although there is considerable variation among them, every state recognizes the patient's right to make fundamental choices about the care and treatment he or she receives at that time.

In all cases—whether you have signed an AMD or not—as long as you retain the capacity to make and express your decisions, your consent must be obtained for your medical treatment. You remain solely and totally in control. If you have an AMD, it can be revoked or modified at any time, if you are capable of doing so.

Although many people have heard of the living will, few realize that this is often a very narrow form of AMD, in terms of the situations it addresses. For example, the living will might only speak about "heroic" life-prolonging measures and might only apply *when death is otherwise imminent.* Such a directive is of no use to the patient who is stable but in a coma with no chance of recovery. Most of us planning along these lines hope to cover all the bases. There are two means to do this: preparing a comprehensive medical directive of your wishes in advance of need, and appointing someone to speak for you on these matters when you cannot.

In most states, a health care *agent, surrogate,* or *proxy* can be selected by the patient. The proxy can be authorized to make any health care decision the patient would have made if he or she had decision-making capacity, as long as it conforms with accepted medical practice. Sometimes this document is called a *health care power of attorney.* Note that the proxy need not be chosen only in anticipation of death. He or she can be empowered to deal with temporary incapacity, too. Of course, you do not have to be a patient before preparing one of these documents.

The AMD can be prepared without an attorney, but you should not just copy an official form and sign it unchanged, unless it reflects what you really want. If available, an official form from the statute books of your state is the best place to start. State-specific guides with sample forms are also available to members of the American Association of Retired Persons (AARP), through its office of Legal Counsel for the Elderly. If you are in a nursing home or other institution, there is generally a patient advocate to consult about making an AMD.

— © Michael T. Palermo, J.D., C.F.P.

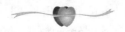

Taking the Financial Worry out of Caring for an Elderly Loved One

Caring for a seriously ill or elderly person can present many challenges. Emotional, physical, and financial stresses take their toll on the patient and everyone involved in his or her care.

There is a little-known way to alleviate financial stress and, although it has been available for more than ten years, many people still are unaware of its existence. I am referring to the option of converting an existing life insurance policy into cash before the insured's death. Once known only as a death benefit paid after one dies, existing life insurance can now be used as a true benefit for life. This option is known as either a *viatical* or *life settlement.* Simply put, the owner of a life insurance policy transfers ownership of it to a third-party funding company. That company in turn pays the insured an amount less than the policy's face value as described below. The seller (the insured, the viator) receives one lump sum payment, and the funding company, now the new owner of the policy, takes over premium payments, and so forth. When the insured dies, the funding company receives the full death benefit directly from the insurance company.

Viatical settlements are designed specifically for people living with a serious or life-threatening illness; life settlements are available for people without a terminal illness, but with a shortened life expectancy nonetheless. For example, generally available for people over age seventy-five, a person who is sixty-five and has significant health concerns may also qualify for a life settlement. A viatical/life settlement specialist must evaluate each case to determine which option is best.

Criteria considered by funding companies include face value, policy type, premium expense, rating of the insurance company, and life expectancy of the insured. Different funding companies have different parameters for policies before they are considered for purchase.

Due to the complexities involved, it is wise to engage the services of an experienced settlement broker, who represents the insured, to present the policy and accompanying paperwork to numerous funding companies. The broker negotiates the highest offer on his or her client's behalf. Aware of the preferences of many funding companies, an experienced viatical/life settlement broker processes an application to completion with no fee. This can save substantial time, energy, and stress associated with such a complex financial transaction. The funding company pays the broker's fee in addition to what it pays the insured.

Life settlement professionals offer viatical and life settlements. Insurance brokers and other financial professionals are not qualified settlement professionals unless they also have proper life settlement licenses.

What you need to know: There may be tax ramifications if you sell a life insurance policy. For example, means-based entitlements may be interrupted. Discuss this with your attorney, accountant, or financial advisor as you would any other important financial transaction.

In some cases other options may exist to obtain cash from a policy. Many life insurance policies now offer a *living* or *accelerated death benefit* (ADB). The percentages paid and the requirements vary. If there is a benefit remaining after the ADB is paid to the insured, it is paid to the beneficiaries. This is an excellent option for people who need extra cash now and who also want to leave money to their loved ones. Older policies may have built up a substantial cash value that can be accessed, or a loan may be available. Term and group insurance policies do not offer these options.

This often-misunderstood industry has experienced dramatic growth in its decade of existence. As the viatical and life settlement industry continues to evolve, so do the regulations and legislation that govern it. Many states have enacted new laws that require all settlement professionals to have specific viatical and/or life settlement licenses. In some states, additional licenses are required, depending on what segment of the industry the company is involved in. The federal government has also taken notice. The Health Insurance Portability and Accountability Act of 1997 (HIPAA) made viatical settlements federally tax free if certain requirements are met.

Bottom line: Do your homework! A life insurance policy is a valuable asset. Knowing your options and investigating them thoroughly will allow for an intelligent decision when selling a policy.

— Carole Fiedler

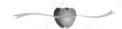

Contractor Hell

Count your fingers, count your blessings, and, for pete's sake, count your money. My mom's house sprang a small leak last summer that expanded into a cross between a Marx Brothers' movie and a modern version of Dante's Inferno.

First, no one could find exactly what was leaking; then the most logical answer by the most competent-looking plumber turned out to be neither logical nor competent. While they were fixing the wrong pipes, the workers loosened the top of the hot water heater and flooded the house. Add nonresponsive insurance agents; slick, slow, and soon invisible contractors; mirror mishaps; and financial chicanery and you have Mom's fall and winter.

Now, when you realize this is happening to a smart woman with involved family members, the number of past and present caregivers open prey to this horror is truly frightening. Please understand that I am not suggesting the vast majority of home improvement specialists fall within this group. They do not. We just got lucky.

Hard-Learned Lessons

Allow me to offer some helpful hints for those with home repair woes:

- Check 'em out! Call the Better Business Bureau and your state to check on any complaints about potential contractors. Talk to previous clients.

- Make sure the contractor has a license. Many times, even if the business is licensed, you never deal directly with the license holder. Make sure that person is aware that you will refer him or her to the proper authorities, if necessary.

- Bid! Bid! Bid! Prices, as well as qualifications, will vary... *greatly.*

- Insist on a time and payment schedule, with penalties for missed scheduled commitments and rewards for beating the schedule with competent work.

- Do not give anyone cash. Never. Not for any reason. Get receipts and, when the work is done, get warrantees.

- Do not pay in advance. If you are asked to pay too much before the work is done, worry.

- Watch the paperwork. Retotal figures. Ask questions. Demand proof. Demand receipts. It is your money, after all.

- Make sure you get *release of liens* from all subcontractors. If you do not, and the contractor fails to pay them, you are liable.

- "If in doubt, don't lay it out!" Get good advice from your attorney if you feel that someone is taking advantage of you.

- Trust yourself. Don't settle for answers that don't ring true.

Now that you've passed Contractor 101, may you never have to take the final exam.

— Gary Barg

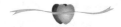

Fight for Your Rights

As a caregiver you must be adept at dealing with insurance issues, especially in today's complicated world of health maintenance organizations (HMOs), preferred provider organizations (PPOs), and long-term care policies. The language alone is enough to send you packing. What happens if your insurer refuses to pay part, or all, of your bills? That's not that uncommon.

What many people don't realize is that they can appeal if their insurer says no. And people who know their rights have an outstanding chance of winning those appeals.

Let's hope you never have to go through that. However, the following are a few suggestions for arming yourself should the need to appeal a refusal of insurance payment arise.

Save everything! Don't discard any insurance papers or any papers pertaining to the patient's treatment. Save receipts for all doctors' visits and all prescriptions. Save copies of referrals to specialists. When speaking with any employee of the insurance company, write down the person's full name, position, extension, and whatever he or she tells you to do. Organizing all of these things in a portfolio can only help.

Make sure the appeal is airtight. Writing a letter defining the patient's position is the first step. A letter is documentation; a phone call is not. The letter should be detailed but concise. Include such important information as the claim number, group number, and policy number. State the reason for coverage denial; then describe the illness and treatment. Next, state why you believe the insurers made the wrong decision and then offer a solution. Close by saying what you would like the insurers to do. The primary care physician and any specialists involved should write letters as well (provided they are on the patient's side).

Keep photocopies of everything sent to the insurer. It is also helpful to keep copies of pertinent medical records. Any procedures that the insurer claims are "experimental or medically unnecessary" should be supported by articles from medical journals.

Obtain the doctor's full support. The primary care physician most likely will stand by the patient through this ordeal. After all, he or she prescribed a drug or recommended a procedure that the insurer doesn't want to pay for. In these cases, the doctor's support is vital to your appeal's success.

So don't take it lying down. Patients have certain rights as insurance consumers. A very small percentage of people ever appeal under these circumstances, but it should happen more. It is probably easier for the insurance company just to pay the claim than to fight it.

— Michael Plontz

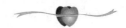

Chapter 3

"Doctor, Can You Hear Me?"

In today's health care system, caregivers must learn to be effective advocates for their loved one and patient, not only with doctors and other health care professionals, but with the insurance and HMO industries as well. In this chapter, you'll hear from experts about some of the issues caregivers must master when dealing with health care professionals.

Top Ten Things a Caregiver Needs from a Health Care Provider

1. **Attention.** The caregiver's loved one may be the twenty-seventh similar case you've seen today, but to the caregiver this is Mom or Dad, sister, or lover.

2. **Compassion.** Be diligent in its application.

3. **Time.** A few moments of your uninterrupted time is some of the strongest medicine you'll ever administer, and it costs so very little.

4. **Respect.** The person pushing the wheelchair is also part-time bookkeeper, psychologist, dietitian, insurance and incontinence expert, and full-time general in the war being waged against this illness. The person not only needs your respect, he or she *deserves* it.

5. **Dedication.** Be relentless in your devotion to your calling. The caregiver has entrusted you with his or her most valuable asset—a loved one. You earn that trust with your skill, knowledge, and ability.

6. **Honesty.** The caregiver is your partner in this endeavor; he or she deserves (and can handle) the truth.

7. **Prudence.** Graceful disclosure of the truth is a true test of a caring professional.

8. **Advocacy.** Never accept less than the best your system has to offer the caregiver's loved one.

9. **Understanding.** The caregiver plays a pivotal role in the well-being of your patient; understanding the needs, wishes, and fears of the caregiver improves your patient's care.

10. **Your well-being.** Know your emotional limit and learn when to ask for help. Your loved ones and the caregiver's loved one need you to remain well.

— Gary Barg

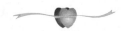

Ten Questions to Ask Your Loved One's Primary Care Physician

1. What exactly is wrong with my loved one?

2. Can you suggest any resources where I might find out everything there is to know about my loved one's condition?

3. Is this condition treatable?

4. What can I expect, or how will the condition progress?

5. What can I do right now as far as caring for my loved one?

6. Do I need any special equipment?

7. Will my loved one have to be on medication?

8. Can you offer the best care for my loved one, or should we seek the help of a specialist?

9. Is this condition hereditary?

10. Is the treatment covered under my loved one's insurance?

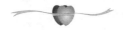

Home Health Care Aides: Establishing a Positive Relationship

You've made the decision to let an aide come into your home to help. That was hard enough. Now you're apprehensive about what to expect when the aide arrives for work. If you don't have experience with in-home assistance, all sorts of "worst-case scenarios" are whirling around in your head. And then there are the questions. What should you do if you don't like the aide? How should you approach problems? Who supervises the aide?

Assuming that you have hired an aide from a home health care agency, you can expect a lot of support in easing your anxieties. It is the agency's job to answer your questions in advance and resolve any issues that arise. The key to facilitating your satisfaction and comfort is good communication with the agency management and with your aide.

Here are a few tips for establishing positive relationships with your home health care professionals:

- Be completely honest about your needs.

- Overcome any embarrassment or guilt associated with describing why you need help and what kind of help you need. Remember that you are dealing with professionals who have helped a variety of clients. They are experienced in meeting the needs of people just like you. Home health care professionals are prepared to deal with tough situations such as Alzheimer's, alcoholism, Parkinson's, strokes, incontinence, and stressful family circumstances.

- State your preferences from the start. The best way to get exactly what you want is to be specific. Give a detailed request to the agency so that the aide it sends will meet your needs. Items to include are your household rules, such as no smoking or kosher kitchen. Be sure to define your daily routines and how to follow them, such as up at 7 A.M., breakfast first, medicine second, shower last; I need privacy from 9 A.M. to 11 A.M.; transportation to salon every Friday, using employee's car.

- Give feedback to the agency on a timely basis. "Nip it in the bud" is good advice. Most problems start out small and can best be resolved when addressed promptly. If you are having a problem with the aide, call the agency. This benefits you in two ways: you do not have to be involved in reprimanding the aide, and it prompts the agency to resolve the problem diplomatically. Employee supervision is the responsibility of the agency. If the problem cannot be resolved to your satisfaction, request that the agency send a different aide. The agency will handle the hiring and firing.

If you start off with honesty and communication, having a home health care aide can be a successful and beneficial experience.

— Kim Champion

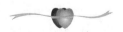

Getting Involved: An Introduction to Rehabilitation

What should a caregiver expect when a loved one is facing a long regimen of rehabilitation? The whole process can be a mystery, and it is often unclear what role the caregiver should play in the process.

The more progress your loved one makes in rehab, the better both of you will feel. The process of rehabilitation is not an easy one, but with your help and support, your loved one will get back the most capability possible.

How do you get the most out of your loved one's rehabilitation? It's just a matter of getting *involved.* Make sure you read about your loved one's condition so you can ask the right questions. Try to understand what your loved one is going through medically. Be familiar with his or her insurance benefits. For example, the "length of stay" in a facility should be discussed with the staff. If your loved one dislikes hospital food, ask dietary staff if you can bring the patient's favorite foods.

In rehab, the doctor orders and discharges the therapy or nursing services. Be aware that nurse practitioners, chiropractors, and physician assistants can also give some orders.

Getting involved may mean a lot of different things, depending on your particular situation, but there are certain basic guidelines you should try to follow.

- **Attend the patient conference.** Usually a patient conference is scheduled that family members can attend. Make sure you can be there. If one is not scheduled, ask that one be arranged. At the conference you will be informed about your loved one's overall medical, physical, emotional, and psychological status. The goals for the patient are established and the expectations of the patient, family, and medical professionals, including case managers, are discussed.

- **Discuss your loved one's progress.** When therapy has started, you should frequently discuss the progress your loved one is making with the physical therapist, occupational therapist, in-house doctor, and nurses. Ask any questions that you have and make certain your perception of how your loved one is doing is similar to theirs.

- **Ask permission to read the medical charts.** Do not be intimidated by the medical setting or your lack of a medical education. Go over every page and ask about anything you don't understand. Remember that everything is written in the medical charts, including changes in medication. The patient has the right to go over his or her chart, as does the primary caregiver with proper authorization. You can ask the case manager for details.

- **Participate in all therapeutic activities.** Attend every activity, including physical therapy (PT), occupational therapy (OT), and speech therapy appointments. Talk with each of the different therapists about your loved one's routine. Family members with appropriate training can learn and do some of the exercises. Ask if you can help do the exercises with your loved one in his or her free time.

- **Encourage your loved one to attend every scheduled activity.** Rehabilitation is never easy, and your loved one will need your support and encouragement to get the most out of it. It also helps the patient battle depression. Success depends in large part on the patient's willingness to get better, but always keep in mind that your loved one has the right to have a bad day or even refuse therapy entirely.

- **Plan for your loved one's homecoming.** When your loved one has shown sufficient progress to think about going home, you should inquire about the discharge date and involve yourself with the planning in plenty of time. Ask about the necessary equipment that Medicare or insurance will pay for. If the equipment cannot be purchased through insurance, go to the nearest secondhand shop or look in the classified section of your local paper. I have seen brand-new walkers, bedside commodes, canes, and wheelchairs for sale at a fraction of their new price. If you do find secondhand equipment, make sure you have it checked with the PT, OT, and nursing staff. Medical equipment shops also offer secondhand items, as do some charitable institutions.

As the primary caregiver, you are an important member of a team working to improve your loved one's health. Your understanding and participation is just as important as that of the medical professionals who are working very hard to improve your loved one's physical and mental outlook. Work with us and ask questions and we will all see the best results.

— Christian Andaya, P.T.

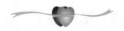

The Caregiver's Role in Rehabilitation

The ever-expanding role of caregivers has grown by leaps and bounds in the last few years, but caregivers have always been extensions of their medical facility–based counterparts, whether they are doctors, physiologists, nutritionists, or psychologists.

The field of rehabilitative medicine is no different. There is a growing need for rehabilitative and therapeutic practice beyond the traditional medical setting. Many health clubs now provide some rehabilitative services once found only in the clinical setting.

Caregivers are also in a unique situation to help administer rehabilitative prescriptions for their loved ones as part of the care team. Effective rehabilitation requires effective communication. Poor communication results in lost time in the rehabilitation process. Caregivers are a vital link between the other health care professionals and their loved one.

Besides maintaining communication, caregivers today may help implement their loved one's exercise program. Part of this program may include actively moving an injured limb through a range of motion, assisting in flexibility exercises, or even applying manual resistance in strengthening activities.

Occasionally you will be asked to become part of the testing and recording of the progress of your loved one. Report writing, exercise logs, updates, contracts, and so forth are all valuable tools for evaluating progress. Make sure all reports are in a legible, orderly format for other health care personnel. Written documentation also can prove invaluable should legal issues arise.

Many caregivers also find themselves in the role of motivator for their loved ones, helping them adhere to their therapy and program. Simply being present can help to keep patients progressing.

For legal reasons, programming decisions must be left to the medical professionals in charge of the case. But the caregiver should question decisions if they don't seem to make sense. Make sure your concerns and those of your loved one are understood and addressed by the health care professionals.

It is equally important that you understand the strategy of the rehabilitative process and not deviate from the medically designed plan. Make sure you are comfortable in this assistance role and feel confident that you have received ample training and supervision for any active role you may play in actual program assistance.

Above all, caregivers must be sensitive to the individual needs of their loved one during the rehabilitative process. Patience and understanding are especially vital in rehabilitative relationships. Caregivers need to be familiar with their loved one's condition, medical terminology, and treatment procedures. This will aid in communication and interactions with medical personnel. The more positive the environment and interactions, the more positive the outcomes.

Rehabilitation Terminology

To help ensure effective communication throughout the rehabilitation process, here are some commonly used terms to describe certain conditions and exercises. This list is in no way exhaustive.

Active-assisted exercise: Exercise in which patients are helped through a range of motion (ROM) that they are unable to do by themselves.

Active exercise: Exercise in which movement is done entirely by the patient.

Closed-chain exercise: Any exercise in which the exercising body segment is attached to a fixed surface such as a floor, requiring the entire limb to bear the resistance—for example, squats for the legs.

Coordination: The working together of various muscles in the execution of movement.

Cross-transfer: A neurological phenomenon in which training the "healthy" limb helps to strengthen the immobilized limb.

DAPRE: Daily adjustable progressive resistance exercise, a program often used in rehabilitation.

Flexibility: Range of motion possible in a joint or series of joints.

Limited ROM exercise: Exercise in which the range of motion is limited due to an injury or the biomechanics of the injury.

Non-weight-bearing exercise: An exercise in which body weight is not borne by the lower extremities.

Open-chain exercise: An exercise in which the end of the exercising body segment is not fixed to the end of a floor, wall, etc., and is freely movable—for example, leg extensions.

Passive exercise: An exercise in which the patient is taken through a range of motion by a therapist, caregiver, or machine.

Reconditioning: Restoration of preinjury or preconditioning levels of physical fitness through a prescriptive therapeutic exercise program.

ROM: Range of motion; the measurement of the range that a limb moves through space around its joint.

Rehabilitation Strategies

Regardless of why your loved one needs a rehabilitation program, the goal of the therapy is to help restore levels of fitness to their preinjury state or better. In cases of chronic illness or disability, programs focus on improving the quality of life and comfort. To achieve this, many techniques are used, depending on the therapeutic goals and objectives.

Before programming begins, however, testing of functional capacity is normally done to establish baselines and future progress. Areas tested can include muscular strength, power, endurance, flexibility, and ROM. Some of the devices used include calipers, isokinetic instruments, goniometers, and dynamometers.

After testing, therapeutic exercise programming and selections begin. The basic program structure allows for a warm-up before activity, reconditioning exercises, then a cool-down period.

Most rehabilitation programs are geared toward progress. In regard to resistance training and strength improvement, one of the most commonly used programs is the DAPRE system. This is a four-set exercise program (the first two sets are progressive warm-ups) that takes into consideration the daily variations in a patient's strength. Resistance can be applied through weights, machines, latex bands, or manually, by the caregiver or therapist.

Another common exercise prescription for strength improvement is isometric exercises. An isometric contraction occurs when the muscle is neither shortened nor lengthened, merely contracted and tensed. Tension is generated, and energy is released in the form of heat, not mechanical work. Pushing against an immovable object such as a wall is an example of isometric exercise. This is especially valuable to a patient who needs to exercise an immobilized limb or when joint motion is hindered by inflammation. Instead of using repetitions to measure work, *seconds of contraction* are the units in isometric programming. Flexibility drills, active-assisted exercise, and limited ROM exercises are also used by the therapist and introduced to the caregiver.

— Sean Kenny, C.P.T.

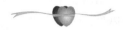

The Medicalization of Personal Needs

Among the many caregiver responsibilities, there are three I wish to address here: those that are medical, those that address personal needs, and those in the gray area in between.

First, let's consider the three categories. Medical responsibilities most often are assumed by physicians, nurses, and other clinicians, but, under special circumstances, the patient or caregiver may take over, at least temporarily. The responsibility for personal needs, such as bathing and feeding, is almost entirely assumed by the patient or the caregiver, except when the patient occupies a bed in a hospital or nursing home.

The gray area of responsibility is the main focus of this piece. Examples include administration of insulin by injection, taking pulse and blood pressure readings, and so on. I predict that we will see a shift in the number of responsibilities from medical and health care professionals to caregivers. Health plans will cover fewer and fewer benefits, and medical responsibility—as defined by those paying for benefits—will be more circumscribed.

When I graduated from medical school in June 1966, I characterized almost any need a patient had as something that should be covered under the patient's health plan. Physicians essentially were able to establish medical necessity by declaration. Another way to look at it is that I participated in an American cultural and social movement to "medicalize" all the needs of patients. If the patient had a need, we construed it as representing a medical necessity.

Medicalization had other origins as well, including an increasing emphasis on public health and preventive medicine. What you ate became a medical matter. Cigarette smoking became a medical matter. Jogging and other exercise became a medical matter. Automobile seatbelts became a medical matter. Within a short period of time—perhaps a decade—medicalization of ordinary personal activities was rampant in America.

This was good for many people. The notion was that anything that had to do with health, well-being, and normal functioning was "medical" and therefore a covered health plan benefit.

With widespread adoption of the managed care mentality, with its emphasis on minimizing expenditures, we've reversed this trend and no longer declare a particular need or consequent service to be "medical." For example, mental health disorders were declared totally separate in terms of medical decision making and financial responsibilities of health plans. If your heart is sick, they'll spend thousands and thousands of dollars. If your brain is sick, maybe a few hundred. Why? Who made these decisions and with what authority?

In the meantime, my focus here is on the increasing exclusion of needs and services that could be attended to or provided by caregivers. One of the most important areas of medical consumer contention that I deal with daily is the denial of payment for services because the services can be provided by a caregiver, even though just a few years ago they were almost automatic health plan benefits. And this pattern is expected to continue with increasing intensity.

Health plans and professional medical groups (which do almost all of the utilization review and denials of health care benefits) are becoming looser in their determination that a patient with a stroke has *plateaued* or merely requires *custodial* care. This simply translates into caregivers (if the patient has them) assuming responsibility for maintaining the patient's health and well-being.

This trend will continue. Caregivers will assume financial and hands-on responsibility for what in the 1960s, '70s, and early '80s was provided for by health plans. One of the ways to prepare for this situation is to be willing to use organizations with names that connote "Caregivers 'r Us," allowing for hiring of people to provide the various services that traditional caregivers provide. Such expenses will be outside the realm of medical necessity and benefits.

Over the long run, caregivers will need to decide whether relegation of such expenses to nonreimbursable costs is appropriate or whether the medicalization of such services is most appropriate. Choose deliberately, choose wisely.

— Vincent M. Riccardi, M.D.

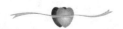

Chapter 4

Care Tips

A Caregiver's Litany

For the day that starts and ends well,
We are thankful.
For medications that work—most of the time,
We are thankful.
For the hand that is steady, the foot that can step,
We are thankful.
For the struggle that ends in success,
We are thankful.
For the smile that cracks the mask,
We are thankful.
For nights of healing rest,
We are thankful.
For shared communication,
We are thankful.
For those who understand,
We are thankful.

For memory of days past, and hope for tomorrow,
for love that sustains us both,
We are, most of all, thankful.

— Camilla Hewson Flintermann

When Thirty Seconds Are Enough

Recently it was my turn to accept attention from caregivers after many years of giving pastoral spiritual care to others. The occasion was a radical prostatectomy. This was the first time I experienced recovery from major surgery.

In those days in the hospital immediately after surgery, I could think only of myself and how my body would deal with the next few minutes of life. Nurses, doctors, and their associates were working hard to keep up with urgent needs of many patients. Family members and friends were coming to visit and doing their best to fit in with the hospital way of life.

In this high-pressure situation, spiritual needs long for attention. People who care deeply bring a spiritual presence that restores one who is working at recovery. However, caregivers may question the value of their efforts in the midst of intense medical activities. My experience says that recovery is given spiritual meaning by the people who come.

Recovery is hard work. It is helpful to think of the energy being expended by all those involved in surgical recovery. The person in the hospital bed who appears to be so quiet is, in fact, working the hardest of all. Intense effort is being spent to reorganize and reassemble a life. The body has been violated, and its defenses and healing mechanisms are put into action.

There is little energy available to respond to staff or visitors. It may appear that the person in the bed is distant, remote, and uninterested in those who come to show their support. Paying attention to a visitor for thirty seconds can seem like an eternity to the one who is on sedatives and unable to move about due to intravenous tubes, catheters, and other devices.

In the midst of the hard work of recovery from surgery, there can be brief moments when caregiving people speak the name of the person in the bed, say their own name, give a word of encouragement, and then leave the room or stay nearby quietly.

Jews and Christians, in particular, speak of such an event as "Sabbath rest." It is reminiscent of the biblical Genesis account of God placing the Sabbath as a day of rest in the creation process. These moments offer the recovering one an opportunity to connect with another person and take a break from overwhelming personal concerns. Spiritual renewal takes its place in the healing of a life.

Such Sabbath rest moments will be remembered and rehearsed by the recovering person when nights are long and sleep won't come. Such brief encounters are a major investment in the health of the one who has undergone surgery. Caregivers can be assured that their presence is an important part of recovery.

The caregiver says, "What shall I say or do?" The recovering person says, "Say my name, say your name, encourage me. Then let me be quiet. My work of recovery continues. Come back again. Thank you."

— Delton Krueger

Taking the Fight out of Mealtime!

At any age, your loved one's eating habits are difficult to control. Witness the two-year-old who will only eat the bun, but no hot dog. Two days later she will eat only the hot dog, not the bun! Or the senior who seems only to pick at a meal, and the teen who thinks a burger and soda provide all the essential nutrients, as long as a chocolate bar is thrown in for good measure!

What can you do? Here are some tips:

- Offer meals with a variety of choices (which you control) and let the care recipient choose how much. A protein source (meat, fish, chicken, or beans); a dairy product (milk, yogurt, or cheese); a starch (rice, potato, peas, corn, or bread); vegetables (from artichoke to zucchini); and fruit (as dessert) will give them choices.

- Put small portions of all the meal items (including dessert) at the place setting at the beginning of the meal. Let your loved one eat in any order. He or she most likely will eat more, even if dessert is eaten first. (A fruit and vanilla low-fat yogurt compote is an excellent dessert choice filled with vitamins, minerals, and protein.)

- Involve your loved one in planning the family dinner as often as possible, but at least once a month.

- As much as possible, let your loved one help with meal preparation. For example, let him or her make fruit salad using a blunt knife or tear the greens for a tossed salad.

- Be sure your loved one is erect and seated comfortably while eating, whether at the table or in an easy chair or bed.

- Provide utensils that support independent ability to feed oneself. Speak to an occupational therapist about special utensils if self-feeding is too laborious.

- Snacks are an important source of nutrients if your loved one eats small meals. Offer foods with lots of protein, vitamins, and minerals.

- Offer water to quench thirst before meals. Drinking juice, fruit punch, or soda will make your loved one too full to enjoy healthy meals and snacks.

- Provide opportunities to engage in physical activities, if at all possible. Exercise builds muscle, naturally stimulates the appetite, and gives a sense of accomplishment. There are exercise videos for use in a seated position, too!

— Rita Miller-Huey, M.Ed., R.D., L.D.

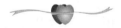

Prescription Medication Safety

More than two million Americans experience adverse drug reactions from prescription medication each year. Patients develop complications from these medications when doctors, pharmacists, and health care professionals ignore precautionary measures and lack communication skills.

Prescription medication safety is crucial for preventing adverse drug reactions or death, and caregivers can become involved in preventing these errors.

Properly prescribing and administering medication means knowing all the facts. Caregivers can prevent allergic, crossover, or adverse drug reactions and overdoses by educating themselves. (Crossover reactions occur when a care recipient takes incompatible medications.) Knowing all the facts includes knowing the medical history of the care recipient and informing the health care provider.

- Be sure to give the health care provider complete medical records. Records can be sent by a previous provider or provided by the caregiver or patient. Medical history records should contain surgeries, immunizations, allergies, and family health history (for example, diabetes, colon cancer). It is also important to notify the health care provider of any social changes, including sleeping patterns, work schedules, and special diets. This will assist the health care provider in choosing a compatible medication.

- Following the directions of the medication is imperative to ensure safety. Read all written materials and instructions carefully. Dispense only the recommended dosage and finish the entire prescription as instructed. All prescribed drugs should have a physician package insert and provide proper labeling. The U.S. Food and Drug Administration requires prescription pharmaceutical manufacturers to offer patients certain information about the drug. This insert should include how to administer the drug safely, possible side effects, and when to take it. Find out if the medication should be taken before or after eating, with a glass of water, and if any food or drink should be avoided. The label also will indicate if any activities, such as driving, should be avoided due to drowsiness while on the medication. If any information is unclear, contact the pharmacy or health care provider.

- There is a possibility of side effects with most prescribed medications. A side effect is a secondary and unusual adverse effect of the drug that may or may not be predicted. These are in addition to the sought-after effect of the medication. Educate yourself on the possible side effects of any prescribed drugs. Many pharmaceutical manufacturers have a Web site or toll-free telephone number where caregivers can get information about a particular drug's side effects.

- After the drug has been administered, it is important to be aware of the care recipient's reaction. Monitoring the care recipient after administering the medication could prevent an overdose or fatality. If symptoms seem unusual or rare, contact an emergency number immediately.

- Never administer prescription drugs in the dark, and be sure to keep them in their original containers to avoid mix-ups with other medications. Monitor expiration dates constantly.

The caregiver and recipient can play a large part in medication risk reduction by communicating openly with health care professionals and pharmacies. Prescription medications are meant to assist in the healing process, but they are not without risk.

— Jennifer B. Buckley
(Information provided by the American Medical Association, Partnership for Patient Safety, and the nonprofit group 21st Century Consumer.)

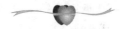

Home Care Tips for Elderly Loved Ones

If you are caring for an elderly loved one at home, you should make him or her as comfortable and safe as possible. This can reduce stress for you and your loved one. The more secure your loved one feels, the less likelihood he or she will become confused, aggressive, or agitated. There are simple, little changes you can make to ensure contentment for your loved one.

1. Buy a small, lightweight pitcher. Keep it filled with water at all times in a convenient place for your loved one. Periodically remind him or her about drinking plenty of water and where the pitcher of water is located. Staying adequately hydrated can ward off a number of different ailments, such as headaches, sleeplessness, and appetite suppression; it's great for overall health and well-being.

2. Avoid placing a lot of mirrors around your home. Mirrors can be confusing for elderly people because they may not recognize their own reflection. Also, walking up to a mirror can startle or confuse them. If you like

to have mirrors in your home, buy smaller ones and hang them relatively high up on the walls to prevent your loved one from seeing his or her reflection.

3. Use large dials and number pads. If your loved one enjoys watching television, buy a remote with large numbers. If your loved one can still use the phone, make sure the keypad has oversized numbers. Also, place digital clocks around your home because they are easier for your loved one to read.

4. Buy your loved one's clothing in basic colors like black, tan, white, cream, and green. This will make it easier for him or her to pick out his or her own outfit. In addition, place all your loved one's shirts on one side of the closet and shorts, pants, and skirts on the other side. Take away any clothes he or she hasn't chosen to wear in a while and keep them in another closet or box.

It is better for your loved one to make as many decisions as possible so he or she feels in control and has a sense of importance. The main thing is to limit choices; too many can be confusing and overwhelming.

— Jennifer B. Buckley

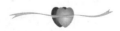

Caregiver's Emotional First Aid Kit

1. Smile; it's not funny how often we forget to do this simple act and how well it lifts our spirits.

2. Call someone who makes you feel good, especially if you haven't spoken with him or her in a long time.

3. Have a bite of something sinfully delicious, while being conscious of your own dietary limitations. When was the last time you treated yourself to a snack?

4. Take a bubble bath, once you make sure that your loved one is safe and secure; nothing expresses caregiver self-care better than a leisurely bubble bath.

5. Read, pick up that novel, or reread that motivating poem. When was the last time you turned off the television, turned down the phone, and read something nice? (This tip goes very well with number 3.)

6. Get a massage. It's like taking a mini-vacation: it will relax you and relieve the tension you build up every day.

7. Buy yourself some flowers. You deserve them, and the sight and smell of something beautiful and fragrant will give you a reason to smile (see number 1).

8. Take a walk at a pace that allows you to feel the wind washing over you.

9. Go shopping and buy something just for you, something that makes you feel special.

10. Go online. You can explore different places, find new friends, and learn new things. Make the Internet your getaway even when you can't get out of the house.

— *Today's Caregiver Magazine*

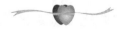

Tips from a Caregiver Husband

My wife, Nikki, suffered a severe stroke in August 1996 that left her partially paralyzed and unable to speak or walk or care for herself in general. She was hospitalized locally for a month and then transferred to a rehab center in Salt Lake City, where she underwent extensive rehabilitation for over a month. After receiving her prognosis from our family doctor, I realized our lives had changed dramatically. It was now up to me to take care of the two of us.

Fortunately, we are both retired and our children are grown and married. We do have two dogs that had to learn along with me. There wasn't much I could do at the local hospital immediately after the stroke except to be with Nikki every moment I could. I was allowed to remain with her throughout the day and night if I desired. In fact, I spent some nights sitting and napping in a chair if she was having a rough time. The doctor and nurses convinced me to go home around 8 P.M. after a few days, but I was allowed to call the nurses' station for a report on her condition before I went to bed. Our sons and daughters came the day after she was hospitalized so we were able to have someone with her at all times. More important, I had support. We limited visitors to family only. The children left ten days later, once her health was steadily improving.

When Nikki was transferred to the rehab center, I made plans to go too. I received permission from the center to park our motor home in its parking lot. The center even furnished me with water and electricity hookups, and I was allowed to use the employees' shower and restroom if I wanted. Living in the motor home was a blessing because I could be with her from 7 A.M. until she went to bed, and dogs could be there, too.

For the first two days, I observed the nurses, therapists, and other rehab personnel to see where I would fit in. By the third day I was helping to dress Nikki, transfer her from wheelchair to bed or chair, and assist in her feeding, which was "family style" in the dining room. I also participated in her physical and speech therapy. Our dogs were allowed, even encouraged to visit with her in her room, or she could be wheeled out to the motor home to visit them.

At times, I felt I was getting in the way by being so nosy and inquisitive, but the doctor explained that the program was as much for my benefit as for Nikki's. I was allowed to take her outside, and after awhile she was allowed passes so we could go out to dinner or visit family in the area.

Our oldest returned for another visit and was surprised when her mother and I were both at the airport to meet her. I received valuable training and information at the rehab center to help me in my role as caregiver. I learned about hospital beds, wheelchairs, ramps, medications, feedings, personal hygiene care, and much more just by observing and asking questions. Nobody ever ignored me or laughed at me; in fact, they all went out of their way to assist me.

When Nikki was discharged, we already had the house partially ready with a hospital bed and riser on the toilet.

The children returned to help. One daughter is a registered nurse, so she was in charge. She will never know how much her help was needed and appreciated. We had home health assistance scheduled for twice a day but soon discovered the morning visit was sufficient. The children stayed until the end of November, celebrating Thanksgiving and Nikki's birthday before they left. The day they left was the day reality hit me like a ton of bricks. I had never felt more alone or afraid in my life. Now it was up to me to cook, clean, do laundry, shop, feed the dogs, you name it. I became very depressed.

Grown men do cry... I went to our doctor, talked and cried in the exam room, and he prescribed medication that has been a blessing to me ever since.

I knew how to wash clothes but had never bothered to learn how to operate our own washer. One of our daughters took the time to teach me. Thank God for wash and wear. Cooking is something a man should not fear. If you can read, you can cook. Follow directions. Frozen dinners aren't too bad either. I made a list of the meals Nikki and I enjoy and pasted it on the cupboard door. When I don't know what to have, I refer to the list for an idea. Don't be afraid to try; the worst that can happen is you'll throw it away and go out to eat. Clean up the kitchen and use the dishwasher if you own one. I keep a good supply of paper plates on hand, too.

Here are a few other tips I have found to be very helpful. Learn how to clean house. Dust, mop, and run the vacuum, and don't forget to empty the bag. Hire somebody for the deep cleaning once a year; it is well worth it. I ask all visitors to telephone first, and an answering machine is very useful when Nikki is in the shower or getting dressed. Also, it is a good idea to install rails in the shower and bathroom, if needed. Remove the showerhead and install a handheld sprayer. Don't forget liquid soap, shampoo/conditioner, and lotion. Oh, yes, and learn how to shave legs.

Personal hygiene is very important. If incontinence is involved, keep a good supply of adult diapers on hand. Don't be afraid to ask a pharmacist or your doctor what kind to purchase. I found that a female clerk is very helpful if you explain your situation. Disposable rubber gloves are a must. Keep a box in the bedroom and bathroom. Here again, ask if you can purchase a few boxes from your doctor; it is a lot cheaper. In our case, my wife needs assistance to use the bathroom, and she is unable to wipe herself after a bowel movement. Keep a supply of disposable baby wipes handy along with a plunger near the commode.

I have a baby monitor in Nikki's bedroom so she can call me during the night when she needs to go to the bathroom. When we are out in public and she needs to use the restroom, I explain the situation to an employee. In all cases the employee has checked the ladies' room for us and kept others out. If someone does enter, I stand outside the stall and let the woman know what is happening, and that it is "true togetherness." Nobody has become upset and some even offer to help. In public areas, such as parks, I ask someone to check out the restroom for us and have yet to be turned down. The helpful stranger usually stands guard outside without being asked.

I have learned how to apply Nikki's makeup and comb her hair. Get to know your loved one's beautician. We have Nikki's hair cut every six weeks. We can go to the beauty salon now, but had to have the beautician come to the house, even the hospital, in the early days.

Learn your wife's clothing size, including underwear. Check the tags for sizes. If uncertain, ask a daughter, daughter-in-law, or anyone else you feel might be able to help. Again, female salespeople can be a big help. Nikki's wardrobe now is mainly sweatpants and sweaters. We have at least two "dressy" sweat outfits for when we go out. Tennis shoes with Velcro straps have replaced heels and boots. Because we are men, we understand how to remove a bra from our teen years. I recommend that you learn how to put one on your spouse. One word of caution: do not attempt to dress her in panty hose. That is an exercise in complete frustration, but it's worth a good laugh in the end. Although Nikki is unable to speak or read and write, we are able to communicate in our own way. We keep laughter in our house.

Make certain your wills are in order, along with powers of attorney, which you will need to sign your wife's name to certain items. Your family attorney can assist you in these matters.

Caregiving is a full-time job, twenty-four hours a day, 365 days a year. I am able to leave the house for at least an hour in the morning and again in the afternoon. I look forward to shopping as I meet people in the stores. Sometimes I just go for a walk. I bought a computer in February to email our children. I know nothing about computers except how to turn them on and off, and I'm not a typist either. I found a whole new experience out there, people whose situations are the same, or in some cases, worse. I look forward to the support I receive from other caregivers. Now the children hear from me once a week, but they are happy and understand the support we caregivers give one another.

I don't look at myself as a caregiver; I am a husband in love with his wife.

— Sandy Senor

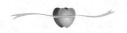

Chapter 5

Caring for Aging Loved Ones

Alzheimer Patient's Prayer

Pray for me; I was once like you.
Be kind and loving to me; that's how I would have
treated you.
Remember I was once someone's parent or spouse,
I had a life and a dream for the future.
Speak to me; I can hear you even if I don't understand
What you are saying. Speak to me of things in my
past to which I can still relate.
Be considerate of me; my days are such a struggle.
Think of my feelings because I still have them and
can feel pain.
Treat me with respect because I would have treated
you that way.
Think of how I was before I got Alzheimer's; I was
full of life,
I had a life, laughed and loved you.

Think of how I am now; my disease distorts my
    thinking,
My feelings, and my ability to respond,
But I still love you even if I can't tell you.
Think about my future because I used to.
Remember I was full of hope for the future just like
    you are now.
Think how it would be to have things locked in your
    mind and
Can't let them out. I need you to understand and
    not blame me,
But Alzheimer's.
I still need the compassion and the touching and
    most of all I
Still need you to love me.
Keep me in your prayers because I am between life
    and death.
The love you give will be a blessing from God and
    both of us will
Live forever.
How you live and what you do today will always be
    remembered
In the heart of the Alzheimer's Patient.

— © Carolyn Haynali

Michael, My Baby Brother

He was a beautiful baby, and, fortunately for my parents,
there was just enough age difference between us that they
had a built-in baby-sitter. And I was thrilled to oblige. We
went to the beach, to the park, on picnics; I loved being
with him. Michael has lived in Reno, Nevada, for the past

few years, so when the call came from the Reno coroner's office, I knew immediately that my baby brother was dead. It came as a cold shock.

It was a call I never expected to receive. Michael was only forty-nine years old. He had died of heart failure. The details were to become clear over the next few days, but one of my first thoughts was how to share the information with my dad, and that I needed his strength and support.

That was when I realized I had suffered two losses, because even though Dad is alive and physically well (thank the Lord), he can't be there to support me. For the moments that he might understand, it would hurt him greatly; and then of course, he would not remember the news moments later. One of the silent losses suffered by having a loved one with Alzheimer's or dementia. The person is there physically, but mostly no longer able to be a confidant or advisor.

How do I tell him that his son has died? Will he remember he had a son? Do I wake his memory to give him back his son for the few moments it will take to tear his son away again? Is it worth the pain he will go through? But how can I not tell my father that his precious son has died? I admit I don't know exactly how to make this decision.

> Michael, I love you and miss you. I know that you are resting in Mom's arms. Sleep in peace, baby brother.
> Your loving sister,
> Monica

— Monica Weiss Barg

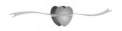

Normal Aging or Dementia?

In the early stages, families and friends find it difficult to distinguish between dementia and normal aging. Initially dementia can be fairly innocuous because most people compensate for minor mental slipups with notes, reminders, and "rational—lies."

Social skills are generally the last to go, so short visits with someone who has early dementia may not reveal anything wrong. She may look as she always did, chat about old times, and socialize as usual. Caregivers, who don't want to believe that something might be wrong, often dismiss inappropriate appearance, changes in behavior, and memory lapses without realizing it.

At some point, however, the problems become more obvious. Dementia begins to interfere with relationships, work, life, and daily tasks. The person might lose a particular skill. For example, an avid crossword puzzle fan may have difficulty filling in the blanks; a pharmacist may not be able to remember the names of the drugs or the dosage on prescriptions to be dispensed.

If you suspect dementia, think carefully about what the person was like before. Although people with dementia react individually and uniquely to the illness, the following are common signs and symptoms of beginning dementia:

- **Short-term memory loss.** Important details of recent events are forgotten frequently and permanently.
- **Self-neglect.** Personal hygiene is neglected, such as mouth care, brushing hair, or wearing the same or soiled clothing.

- **Erratic emotional responses.** The person becomes more anxious, restless, or tearful.
- **Speech difficulty.** One word is confused for another; finding the right word is more difficult.
- **Impaired abstract thinking.** Counting and balancing the checkbook becomes increasingly challenging, and the person may pay bills twice or forget to pay some at all; a lifetime golfer may have more difficulty choosing the appropriate club.
- **Poor judgment.** The person makes unsafe or unusual decisions. He or she may not remember to make sure traffic is clear before driving or walking across the street.

If caregivers suspect dementia, the family should consult a geriatric doctor and a psychologist or social worker for a possible diagnosis. This hunch may be wrong. If not, keep in mind that at least 5 percent of all cases of dementia are partially reversible. The sooner they are diagnosed, the sooner and more easily they can be treated.

Nestor Galvez-Jimenez, M.D., neurologist with the Department of Neurology at the Cleveland Clinic in Florida, explains that overmedication, adverse drug reactions, vitamin B deficiency, and thyroid gland disorders are some of the reversible causes of dementia. He explains that in the elderly, depression can also mimic the early phases of dementia, causing a disorder known as *pseudodementia.*

If the illness cannot be cured, symptoms often can be treated, including teariness, sleeping problems, and anxiety. A diagnosis forces the family to face the situation and plan for the future while the loved one can still be part of the planning. Learning the biological reasons for a loved one's behavior can increase patience, empathy, and tolerance. Acknowledging overwhelming and harsh realities may be extraordinarily painful, but it is the only way to move forward.

— Sherri Issa, L.C.S.W., M.S.W., D.A.B.C.M.

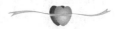

Alzheimer's: Altered Perceptions

Most of us are familiar with the phenomenon in which an Alzheimer's patient does not recognize his or her own reflection any more—either in a mirror or in a car window. Because brain cells are dying out and not being replaced, patients do not actually know whom they are looking at. Think of the brain as a computer system with "glitches" caused by lack of blood flow to the brain. Different areas of memory are affected; even entire years are completely erased. So, for the typical Alzheimer's patient, the past becomes the present—while the present becomes the future.

This means that such patients are living in the past, where their brain cells are still alive, alert, and functioning. This may be at age seventy, sixty, fifty, or even farther back. But this becomes their present, their actual reality. It is as if suddenly we were transported twenty-five years ahead in our own lives, into the future. We would be just as lost, confused, terrified, and irritated as they are.

They do not understand their futures any more than we would. We would not recognize ourselves as old people either. I remember showing my mother a mirror and her telling me that "she looked like an old lady"; she did not know who she was. I showed her picture albums and she knew herself up to the age of fifty. All images of her after that time were completely foreign to her, erased in her own memory banks never to be retrieved.

It is my strong opinion that we, the caregivers of the Alzheimer's patient, should try to function in the patient's reality, which is in his or her past, wherever the brain is still alive, alert, and functioning. Rather than trying to impose our time on them, it is far easier for us to enter their time temporarily, listening to the memories they pull from their vast storehouse of information and experiences—whether it be twenty years ago or longer. We can learn a lot from their recollections, because the brain remembers things in vivid detail.

The alternative is to argue with and cajole such people to live in our reality, in a future they do not understand, which is either a nightmare or a dream they cannot make sense of. Arguments ensue, feelings are hurt, and confusion reigns. It takes so little for us to step into their shoes and look through their eyes, live in their reality—if only for a little while. And it is so much less exhausting than trying to force them to live in our reality, just so that we can feel more secure. After all, it is the patient's welfare we are trying to protect and develop, not our own.

I know a lot of people fear that their loved one will some day not recognize them, and they are not sure how they will handle the pain of suddenly being a nonentity. But when my mother no longer recognized me, it was not the saddest part of her illness. Rather, it was when she no longer recognized herself—the things that had brought her great joy and the pleasure she took in living were gone, and her personality was disintegrating, bit by bit, until little else remained.

I do have one memory that stands out during those years of caring for my mother. After having a major stroke and being in a coma for a few days, my mother suddenly woke up. She found herself in the hospital bed in our home, and for some reason her mind had gone back to the time when she was hospitalized for my birth.

I came into the room, and she asked me who I was. I told her my name, and she said, "My, I just named my own daughter that name." I looked into my own mother's eyes and she was literally glowing with joy and pride. I knew I had discovered a secret not many children will ever have the opportunity to witness or grasp—that moment of birth when your own mother is totally in rapturous awe at the thought of you coming into her life. At that moment, looking into her glowing eyes, I knew what I had longed to know my entire life—that I was truly loved, wanted, and desired. My mother loved me! It was like being given a personal glimpse into a past I could never enter otherwise, and what I found was great joy and beauty. I will never forget the glow of love my mother carried for me on my birth.

So, in closing, think about how Alzheimer's patients have experienced a totally altered reality. Their perceptions are altered forever. As the disease progresses, they lose more active brain cells and retreat further back into their memories, into the lives they once lived. This is not like a memory to them now. It is an actual living reality. And once in a great while we get the unique privilege of a glimpse inside their minds, their hearts, their very souls. What we find there is not chaos or turmoil. Instead we find great joy and love in great abundance. We find the beauty of the soul.

— © 1999 Dorothy Womack

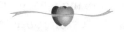

Caring for an Elder from Far Away: Geriatric Care Managers

Balancing work and elder care can be a challenge, whether your parent lives next door or out of state. Add children to this, and the situation is compounded. Legal, financial, and long-term planning for elder care is crucial, and long distance caregivers need to prepare for travel and time off from work. Face the facts: many older adults want to stay where they are. They do not want to relocate, even if it means being closer to family. If this is what the elder wishes, as the child, you must respect that wish.

For people who work and care for an aged family member (particularly when that family member lives far away), one solution is to hire a professional geriatric care manager. A professional geriatric care manager specializes in assisting older people and their families with long-term care arrangements. Care managers have a minimum of a bachelor's degree or substantial equivalent training in gerontology, social work, nursing, counseling, psychology, or a related field.

Prolonged illness, disability, or simply the challenges of aging can alter the lifestyle of older adults significantly. Daily responsibilities can become difficult. Efficient coordination of medical, personal, and social service resources can enhance the quality of life for older adults and their caregivers.

Geriatric care managers assist older adults in maintaining their independence at home and can ease the transition to a new setting. Geriatric care managers also help:

- conduct care planning assessments to identify problems, eligibility for assistance, and need for services;

- review financial, legal, or medical issues and offer referrals to geriatric specialists to avoid future problems and conserve assets;
- act as a liaison to families at a distance, making sure things are going well and alerting families to problems;
- assist with moving an older person to or from a retirement complex, assisted living facility, or nursing home; and
- offer counseling and support.

How do you know when it is time to call a professional? Look for the following signs.

- Is your loved one losing weight for no known reason?
- Does he or she fall?
- Is the home unkempt and becoming unsafe?
- How are meals made?
- Who pays the bills?
- Is the person able to (and does he or she) maintain a neat appearance?
- Has drinking become a problem?
- Is it safe for your parents to drive? If not, who does the driving for them?
- Has there been a sudden memory loss or increased confusion?

—Terry Weaver, M.P.S., N.H.A., C.M.C., A.C.C.

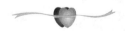

Hydration in Elders: More than Just a Glass of Water

When the weather is warm, it is more important than ever to drink enough fluids. This is particularly true for children and for people aged sixty-five and older, which could be both the caregivers and the care recipient. Not drinking enough fluids can cause unwanted symptoms, complicate existing disease conditions, and account for many hospitalizations of the elderly.

Water and juices are the best; coffee, tea, and colas with caffeine as well as alcoholic drinks cause the body to lose fluids and are recommended only in small amounts.

Elders are at risk for dehydration for many reasons:

- Age: The elderly have less water in their bodies, their kidneys have to work harder to maintain fluid balance, and they often feel less thirsty than younger people.

- Disease-related reasons for dehydration range from the complex to the simple: Infections such as pneumonia, chronic obstructive pulmonary disease, and urinary tract infections increase the need for fluids due to fevers and overproduction of mucus. Some diseases, such as congestive heart failure, renal disease, stroke or other neurological disorders, and diabetes, cause changes in the function of various hormones that regulate the fluid balance in the body.

- Acute reasons for dehydration include prolonged vomiting or diarrhea, overly aggressive diuretic therapy, and poor compliance with medication regimens.

- Environmental: Those with arthritis, diminished vision, or on bed rest have decreased mobility and cannot meet their own needs as easily. Those with diminished appetite or reluctance to bother others for something as simple as help in getting a sip of water are definitely at risk.

- Medications: Some medications may cause increased fluid loss through the kidneys. Diuretics, sedatives, and laxatives are common, necessary drugs that require close attention to fluid intake. Other drugs and alcohol can cause the kidneys to work harder and may damage them, making it harder to maintain fluid balance.

- Psychosocial: Some elderly people are cognitively impaired and possibly unable to drink without full assistance, or may restrict fluid intake intentionally in the hopes of decreasing the risk of incontinence.

- Economic: Some elderly people lack the financial resources to maintain nutritional and fluid intake, extreme or prolonged weather fluctuations, and the possibility of abuse.

How can you tell if your loved one is becoming dehydrated? Consider the risk factors mentioned above. If your loved one complains of nausea; is lethargic; has headaches, vomiting, or dizziness—these could all be signs of dehydration. Call your doctor if your loved one has any or all of these symptoms.

Keep track of how much your loved one actually drinks in a day. A simple way to do this is to put two quarts of water in the refrigerator first thing in the morning, and take all of your loved one's fluids from this container. By the end of the day, at least half of a two-quart pitcher should be consumed. It could take the form of plain water, water with lemon, or other fruit juices made with water.

Regular tea and coffee do not count because they promote fluid loss. Decaffeinated teas and coffees are acceptable (if your loved one will not drink plain water or juices) because they are less likely to promote urination. Foods that melt at room temperature, such as gelatin or ice cream, also have a lot of water content. Serve foods with sauces, juices, and gravies—every little bit helps.

With some conditions it is not appropriate to offer so many fluids: congestive heart failure, cirrhosis of the liver, and kidney disease. However, for most of us, young and old, the rule of thumb is to drink, drink, drink to keep the body hydrated and stay away from the hospital and all the tubes and therapy needed if dehydration does occur.

— Rita Miller-Huey, M.Ed., R.D., L.D.

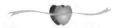

Is It Time to Take Away the Keys?

Caring for a loved one requires walking a fine line. We want our loved one to maintain as much freedom as possible while staying as safe as possible. Keeping the previously mentioned goals in mind, one of the most difficult decisions to make is whether to let your elderly loved one drive.

According to the Insurance Institute for Highway Safety, twelve states now require that older drivers renew their licenses more often than younger drivers. In Illinois, drivers seventy-five or older must take a road test each time they renew. Also, they must renew every two years starting at age eighty-one, and annually after age eighty-seven. A similar bill proposed in California last year was labeled "ageist" by its opponents. Ultimately the references to age were deleted.

One thing remains certain. It is not an easy subject to approach with a loved one, but concern for the person's safety is paramount. The main concerns for older drivers are cataracts, decreased reaction time, and loss of peripheral vision. There are operations to correct vision problems, and reaction times also can be improved. Computer training sessions on making quick driving decisions can improve reaction times sometimes by 40 percent or more. These programs are not widely available yet, but others are. The 55 and Alive class given by AARP helps sharpen seniors' driving skills.

However, there comes a time when most loved ones must be persuaded to give up their car keys. While some give them up easily, most need persuasion. If more drastic measures are needed, social workers, police officers, and the Department of Motor Vehicles may be enlisted to help by filing a hazardous driver report. DMV will revoke the license, and most people will comply (though some with bitterness). This approach may appeal to the loved one's respect for authority figures.

This is by no means an easy issue, but when the safety of your loved one is at stake, you have to pull out all the stops.

— Michael Plontz

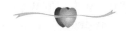

Don't Lose Your Loved One: Alzheimer's and Wandering

If you are a caregiver for a loved one with Alzheimer's, wandering is a major concern. It is a scary proposition for caregivers and a dangerous one for the loved one. We want to give our loved ones all the freedom and independence they can handle while keeping them as safe as possible.

Wandering is common in people with dementia. It causes them to stray or become lost, even in familiar surroundings. What can you do about this problem?

Locks and alarms seem to be the best way to alert caregivers about a loved one's attempts to leave home. The tricky part is assessing your loved one's needs. Each situation is different. People with Alzheimer's change from day to day and stage to stage. What works for one person may not work for another.

Locks may seem a bit inhumane. We are locking our loved one in his or her home or room, but, in case of an emergency, is there an exit? Is it better to keep the door locked, for safety, or unlocked, in anticipation of an emergency?

You will have your answer the first time your loved one strays and you can't find him or her. Your loved one may decide to go out for a walk, or just onto the front porch to get the mail. He or she may turn around, not recognize the home, and start wandering in search of the home.

It seems obvious, but one of the best ways to keep someone from wandering is the effective use of locks. You must begin by evaluating all of the exits in your home: windows, sliding glass doors, garage doors, and conventional doors. It may become necessary to install locks on all openings, not just the conventional doorways.

Install the locks in a place where your loved one will not see them. It will be harder to unlock them, and you don't want the person to feel imprisoned, which could trigger an episode fraught with anger and upset. Tunnel vision is a symptom of the disease, so place locks in the upper or lower corners of windows and doors.

It may be necessary to install two locks on each opening. Opening one lock may not be a challenge for some Alzheimer's sufferers, especially those in early stages of the disease. You may even use two different kinds of locks to make it more difficult. You will have to choose the lock(s) that are best suited to your situation.

You may find that you also need to install alarms on some of the openings. As with locks, there are several options open to you. The least expensive and simplest alarm is a set of sleigh bells or jingle bells. Some of these respond to the slightest vibration. As long as you are within hearing range, they are effective. Also, if you have an alarm in your home already, you may be able to have it modified to alert you when motion is detected or windows and doors are being disturbed. Of course, you will have to have the alarm sound toned down. The regular sound will shake everyone up, and it may cause an adverse reaction in your loved one with Alzheimer's.

These approaches may or may not work for you, but one thing that can be an important resource is to register your loved one with the Alzheimer's Association Safe Return Program. For a $40 registration fee, you get an identification bracelet or necklace and iron-on clothing labels, a Caregiver Checklist key chain, a lapel pin, stickers, a refrigerator magnet, and wallet cards. In the event that a loved one wanders away, Safe Return will fax the vital information and photograph to local law enforcement. If a registered loved one is found, the toll-free number on the bracelet or necklace can be called. You can register by phone at (888) 572-8566. The photo will have to be mailed.

— Michael Plontz

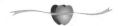

Bathing Someone with Memory Loss

Whether the person with a memory loss is living at home or in a nursing facility, bathing often provokes agitation and distress. It is one of the most stressful tasks faced by caregivers and recipients alike. One of my clients, who lives in a condominium, has a live-in caregiver because of her memory loss. Mrs. Jones (not her real name) is very sweet and easygoing—until it comes time for her bath.

Thankfully, behavioral techniques that we developed and implemented have nearly eliminated the stress of bathing for Mrs. Jones and her caregiver. But it was not always that way. When I first met Mrs. Jones, I was surprised to learn that her neighbors had called the police on two occasions because her screams were so loud. The entire complex knew when Mrs. Jones was having her bath.

It is not uncommon for persons with dementia (memory loss) to resist entering a shower or tub verbally and physically. Why do they resist? In institutional settings, it is common for residents to be undressed in their room by someone they perceive to be a stranger. Remember that the resident suffers from dementia. The caregiver may have cared for this resident for three years, but to the memory-impaired resident, the caregiver is a stranger. Wouldn't you resist if a stranger were taking your clothes off?

Next, the caregiver puts a flimsy gown on the resident, places him or her in a chair with wheels, and pushes the person down the hall with strangers on either side, staring. As the resident enters the shower, he or she may begin to scream because the tiles and faucets are reminiscent of the gas chambers in Auschwitz. The memory-impaired resident perceives that he or she is being taken to the gas chamber.

We unknowingly contribute to the agitation and distress experienced by our loved ones and residents with dementia. Our behaviors play a major role in whether the task of bathing the memory-impaired is successful (that is, not stressful). Caregivers can reduce physical aggression and other agitated behaviors when bathing persons with dementia.

Let's first look at why we bathe. Often when I am in a long-term care facility, and I observe a resident who is not happy about being bathed (this is a very nice way of saying that the resident is agitated), I ask the caregiver, "Why are you taking Mr. Smith to the shower?" Usually, I am told, "Because it is Monday." Or, "Everyone is bathed on Monday, Wednesday, and Friday."

That should not be the reason that you are bathing Mr. Smith! You are bathing Mr. Smith for one of two reasons: Either he has soiled himself and he needs to be cleaned, or he smells—*not* because it is Monday.

Bathing is such a routine part of everyday life that it seems preposterous to ask why we do it. However, when residents and loved ones become distressed by the experience of being bathed, it is worth asking whether, when, how, and how often this has to happen. *Focus on the person, not the task.*

— Terry Weaver, M.P.S., N.H.A., C.M.C., A.C.C.

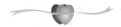

Elderly People May Withdraw to Escape Loss

In the Alzheimer's wing of the nursing home, ninety-three-year-old Ellie Turner stuffs more napkins into her worn-out black purse. The tarnished gold clasp clicks into place for the one hundredth time in one hour. "I have to fix the Underwood," she says as she moves toward the bathroom to change her pants.

Mrs. Turner is called Alzheimer's demented, but I have found that her behavior—and the behavior of thousands like her—makes sense. Her behavior is caused not only by damage to her recent memory, her logical thinking, and her inability to tell clock time, but also by the way she has lived her life. If someone enters her world, accepting or validating her needs, she will not become one of the living dead. She will die with dignity and self-respect.

As a bookkeeper and file clerk for a large electric company, Mrs. Turner used an Underwood typewriter for fifty years. When she was retired against her will at the age of sixty-five, she put her trusty office companion in her dining room. Every morning Mrs. Turner's daughter found her typing for her "company."

Mrs. Turner knew she was retired, but she could not accept the reality of her situation. Her work was the most important thing in her life, and she could not give it up. When, at age ninety-three, she could not accept the fact that she was losing bladder control, she associated the loss of her Underwood with the loss of control. She went to the bathroom to fix her machine. The Underwood became a symbol of her old-age losses.

Very old people who have not prepared for the physical and psychological blows of aging often use symbols to express their needs. They have not learned to face pain, anger, frustration, shame, or guilt. Throughout life, they have denied painful emotions. In very old age, the denial worsens, and they blame others for their own failures.

Each age has its own, unique tendencies. A three-year-old who talks to an imaginary playmate is not hallucinating; she is developing her imagination and verbal skills. If, at age thirteen, she talked to an imaginary playmate, we would worry.

By the same token, an eighty-five-year-old is very different—physically, socially, and psychologically—from a seventy-year-old. We lose thousands of brain cells each year, beginning in our late twenties. Not surprising, this loss of brain tissue can affect our logical thinking areas after eight to ten decades of wear and tear.

Many autopsies have uncovered Alzheimer plaques and tangles in brains of very old people who were never diagnosed with dementia.

Many very old people, eighty-five to one hundred, are interested in the outside world. They have learned to roll with the punches of aging; they do not hang onto outworn roles. They accept what they cannot change.

But there are many very old people who have never learned to deal with their losses or their emotions. Now, in very old age, they cannot face the loss of memory, job, mobility, or control. These are the people who must now look inside. Their job is not to know the outside world. In their old age, they are simply preparing for their final move. They no longer care about the present.

Caregivers can help these people communicate their feelings and put past issues to rest. Rather than viewing them as diseased, we can see them simply as very old people in their final life struggle.

When we tune into their inner world, we begin to understand that a retreat into personal history is a survival strategy, not mental illness. Then we are better prepared to listen with empathy rather than frustration when they step away from reality.

This is validation therapy—a tested method that can be used by both professionals and family members. I developed the therapy in 1963 when, as a social worker, I became frustrated with traditional, reality-oriented approaches to dealing with confused elders age eighty and older. Since then, it's become state of the art and has been embraced by more than three thousand agencies nationwide.

For three decades, validation therapy has helped the very old restore the past, relive good times, and resolve past conflicts. In doing so, it has reduced their stress, enhanced their dignity, and increased their happiness and sense of well-being.

— Naomi Feil, M.S., A.C.S.W.

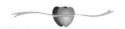

Living with Alzheimer's: "It's Like a Roller Coaster Ride"

— An Interview with Linda Dano

Linda Dano is an acclaimed actress of daytime television. Her talents have brought her an Emmy award for Outstanding Lead Actress for her work in 1993. She sits on the board of directors of Heartshare Human Services. She serves as honorary chairperson for National Alzheimer's Association, works with the National Osteoporosis Foundation, and is the cohost of FFANY Shoes On Sale, an annual event that raises millions of dollars for breast cancer research.

Gary Barg: How did you become a caregiver?

Linda Dano: I'm originally from California; when I moved to New York twenty-two years ago my mother and father remained in California. In the early 1990s my mother began telling me that my dad was forgetting things and acting differently. Eventually, it got to the point where it was becoming exceedingly difficult for my mother to handle my father, but we still had no idea it was Alzheimer's disease. My dad was "cranky," his increasing forgetfulness would make him really angry—angry in a way that wasn't like him. So, my husband, Frank, and I both decided to ask my parents if they could come to New York and live with us.

GB: When were you told that the diagnosis was Alzheimer's disease?

LD: On Thanksgiving morning my father fell. We thought he had broken his hip because he was screaming in pain. At this point he wasn't talking, he was only babbling and yelling—he was completely out of control. After the fall, we got him admitted to Mt. Sinai Hospital, but because his hip wasn't broken and he was still very agitated, the only place they could put him was the psychiatric ward. Still, no one, not one doctor, suggested that my dad might have Alzheimer's.

My dad hated the psych ward. After being admitted he stopped eating and I was told that I should give him a feeding tube. I did because I didn't know what else to do. They told me that we couldn't possibly keep him at home, he was too strong and he was becoming increasingly violent. At this point I met Dr. Robert Butler, head of geriatrics at Mt. Sinai. Dr. Butler was, and still is, at the forefront of Alzheimer's disease research and treatment. It was Dr. Butler who got my dad out of the psych ward and helped me admit him to an appropriate nursing home in New York City... something I swore I would never do.

GB: You must have been devastated. How did all this affect you?

LD: At first I really went in blinded because I didn't want to believe it. How could my father have Alzheimer's? Then, when the diagnosis did come, I was relieved to know that there was a reason for my dad's behavior, and that he wasn't crazy. It was the most traumatic experience of my entire life, watching my dad every day get further and further and further away from us.

GB: What were the things that provided your greatest support back then?

LD: My husband's support and the fact that I was able to save my mother in the process. Had my mother dealt with my father alone away from me, I'm not sure she would have survived. I think it would have taken her down along with my dad. By bringing my mother to be with me in New York I truly believe that I saved her. I'm so thankful for that.

GB: What suggestions do you have for people getting into the same situation?

LD: I believe that people must have a third ear and a third eye when looking at their loved ones—you need to look for warning signs. If you have elderly parents and grandparents, you need to REALLY look at them, don't write off changes in behavior or memory as a normal part of aging. If they're starting to behave differently, you need to have them checked out to see why. You need a proper diagnosis because until you do, you don't know what you're dealing with and you can't put together a plan. You don't overreact. You don't react in a hysterical way, which is what I did. You know what to do.

GB: It seems like one of the biggest challenges for an Alzheimer's caregiver is watching a loved one's mind just slipping away, it's not like cancer or anything else where the mind is . . .

LD: Is still there. You keep hoping there's some little glint in their eye that they know you. One Sunday night, I came in from Connecticut to the nursing home and my father was in bed. It was about 10:00 at night and I patted his face and I said, "Hi, Poppa," and he opened his eyes and he said, "Hi, Linda." It was all that I could do not to get him dressed and take him home. It was the only time he ever said my name where I really believed he knew it was *me* . . . just for an instant, and then it went away again. I cried over that for days.

GB: Once you accept the fact that the person is gone from you and something happens and they're able to come back for a few seconds, it's really a tough . . .

LD: It's like a rollercoaster ride.

GB: That's a perfect way to put it. Did you go to a support group?

LD: No. I didn't do any of it. I just lived with my own pain and I didn't talk about it to anybody. I wasn't making good decisions. I was so guilt-ridden that I didn't go and get information. What was the point? My father had already left me—that was my thinking. I couldn't save him now. I just ate and beat myself up and cried. I never, ever went to the nursing home that I didn't sit on the back staircase and weep before I'd go home.

GB: What are the lessons learned?

LD: We can't let feelings of guilt overtake us. We have to give ourselves a break. As a caregiver you have to also take care of you. You have to reach out for help and you have to ask for help from anyone you can. You need to get into a support group. You need to share. You can't lose you in the process, you just can't. How can you really take care of someone else if you don't take care of yourself? You can't be strong for somebody else if you're a mess.

GB: What are you doing now with regards to Alzheimer's or caregiving?

LD: I've started an educational campaign with the National Family Caregiver's Association. We're offering a package called the "Caregiver Survival Kit." By calling 1-877-439-3566 you'll get the free kit being underwritten

by Novartis Pharmaceuticals. The kit has written information and an educational video about Alzheimer's
disease diagnosis, treatment, and caregiving. I'm also
going to tell my whole story on the Internet so people
will know that they're not alone. I know that there are
many people out there going through just what I did;
my hope is that others will reach out and try and get
the help that I should've gotten myself. I'm quite passionate about this because I know how all-consuming
caring for a loved one with Alzheimer's can become.
Often we're so busy trying to save someone we love
that we lose ourselves in the process. I'd like others to
know that they mustn't do that, for their own sake
and for the sake of their loved ones.

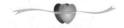

Who Are You?

"Who are you?" he looked at me and asked with
    widened eyes.
Well, I'm your wife of many years—don't act as
    though surprised!!
He studied me again, and said: "Who are you?"—
    Don't delay
I do not recognize a thing in all you've had to say...

Do you come here to take my hand and care for me,
    so dear—
Or are you around to frighten me and cause my heart
    to fear?

I looked at him, this man I'd known for almost all my
   life—
The man who'd raised two children—worked hard,
   and loved his wife.

Within his eyes, I saw the truth—no longer could he
   hide—
He really doesn't know me now although I'm by his
   side!!
I ask for God to strengthen me for all which lies
   ahead—
To heal the stabbing pains I feel inside my heart and
   head.

I'd always thought the cruelest words to one, could
   ever be said
were: "I don't love you anymore"—but I found out
   instead
the hardest words to ever hear—that break your heart
   in two . . .
Are not born out of cruelty . . . but innocence—
And ask: "Who are you?"

— © 1999 Dorothy Womack

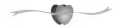

Chapter 6

Specialized Caregiving

Roses Are Blooming

Roses are blooming everywhere
There are beautiful gardens, golden stairs
Trees of every sort and design
All that you ever wanted you find.

Right here in God's Heaven—I'm certain that He
Designed all this beauty, so that all could see
How wondrous His Mercies and Goodness extends
To all who would seek Him—He calls us all Friends.

And He makes a Place where we truly know
That God is within us—and one day, we'll go
Back to all this beauty, surrounded by Him
Where there is no heartache, suffering, or sin
We find all the blessings not known to man
He crowns us with Glory—This Great One—"I AM"
So please don't be saddened, despondent, or grim
For ROSES ARE BLOOMING—And I dwell with HIM . . .

— © 1999 Dorothy Womack

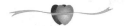

Lincoln's Tears

We came from everywhere. From across the nation, across the continent, around the world. It seemed like we were millions. We came not only to mourn the too early deaths of friends and colleagues and loved ones. We came, all of us, to celebrate life. To celebrate the lives that have fallen victim to AIDS and to those who survive. We came to celebrate the lives of those fighting just to stay alive, and of those who fight for every life.

And we came to honor love. We came to honor the love embodied in The Quilt, which puts our hearts and thoughts and pain and joy on display. The Quilt puts all of humanity touched by AIDS on display. The Quilt may never be seen this way again. It has grown too large to be contained in one place. Its size, the size of its meaning, the enormity of its impact on the hearts and minds of those in its presence has become too large, too vast to be contained in one place. Not even the grandeur of our nation's capital will be able to contain The Quilt in its entirety. The magnitude of it was accentuated by the continuous stream of celebrities and sports figures, politicians, and ordinary citizens, the people reciting an endless list of those who died from AIDS. They read the names every day, morning 'til night. And still, they ran out of time before they ran out of names.

We held our candles high: thousands of candles and hearts, burning brightly in the dark of night, as we marched from The Quilt, which covered the Mall. We marched behind grand marshal Elizabeth Taylor, who led us to the steps of the Lincoln Memorial. Surrounding the Reflecting Pool, we stood, an endless sea of lights. Shining lights, twinkling lights, like a sea of distant stars come to earth to share the love and try to understand.

We stood side by side, and we listened, in the shadow of the Memorial chiseled with words that brought our nation together once before. We listened to speakers, famous and unknown. People who spoke of living with AIDS. One by one they walked out to the podium set high on the steps of the monument, each starting with the phrase, "I am the face of AIDS." White, black, brown, yellow, and red, young and old, male and female, they spoke.

And then she came before us. She took her position on the stage, as in life, with confidence. She stood there, with the great stone figure of Lincoln behind her, facing the inspiration of the Washington Monument, which could only be built when the citizens of this nation pulled together for its common cause. Before her loomed the Capitol, where people who could affect her very survival worked each day and probably never knew until now that she existed. And she faced us, a vast sea of twinkling lights. The strength of her commitment and the power in her presentation defied her age, her frailty. "I am the face of AIDS. I am living with the HIV virus." Her name is Precious, and she is four years old.

As Precious spoke, it occurred to me that while she was looking down at thousands of candles held high, she saw more than just the candles. She saw you and me and my mom and every person who dares to care for any person with any illness, in any pain. For her, the sea of light was the warmth and brightness of those who care, as much as it was a sea of remembrance for those who need our care. The tears we shed did not wash away the flame. Instead it grew into the brighter light of encompassing love and unification within the masses that stood listening to the words of the tiny figure before us.

Beyond Precious I could see Lincoln's strong and benevolent face. I wondered if he understood how the Union he loved so dearly could stand by in silence for so long. Did he understand why the people of his nation did nothing as their children, their sons and daughters, died of AIDS? Did it break his heart, as it breaks the hearts of those who do care, those who do fight, those who won't give up? When Precious ended her speech, I looked again into the face of Lincoln, and I could swear I saw a tear roll down his cheek.

— Gary Barg

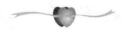

Hope: The Most Caring Gift

In AIDS caregiving, the most caring gift is hope. In my twenty years as a pastor and chaplain, and my fifteen years as a person living with AIDS, I have repeatedly seen the strength, joy, and empowerment that hope brings.

Through my work as a chaplain, I have come to realize that hope is necessary for every person's life, whether we are living with a life-threatening illness or working as caregivers. Hope is important to our own self-care. Hope is also important in maintaining an environment of hope for those we care for. For all of us, hope is an essential ingredient to the quality of life, as long as life lasts.

I survived AIDS, Kaposi's sarcoma, and lymphoma back in the early 1980s, a time when few people survived AIDS beyond two years. First diagnosed in 1982, I lived through two kinds of cancer, hepatitis, CMV, pneumonia, Epstein-Barr virus, valley fever, candidiasis, a variety of fungal infections, herpes, shingles, adrenal insufficiency, neuromuscular problems, peripheral neuropathy, and wasting syndrome. My cancers went into remission in 1985 while I was on an experimental drug, suramin. I got well in 1986. With today's treatments, I now have an undetectable viral load and a CD4 count that hovers around 900. I am "clinically well in all respects," according to my physician, Dr. Alexandra M. Levine.

Hopelessness is a natural reaction to a diagnosis of a terminal or life-threatening illness. Hopelessness happens when we feel helpless to do anything about our situation. Hope happens as soon as we begin to discover how to help ourselves. Despair is passive. Hope is active. Hope happens when we take responsibility for our lives and act.

Dr. Levine gave me hope by inspiring me to act. She made me realize that if I was going to have any chance of survival, I had to stop lying around being depressed and start the work of healing. My mission was to stay alive long enough for science to find a way to manage the disease.

She said I should think of myself as her partner in medicine; we are co-creators of my wellness. Even though there were no treatments, she taught me that I could do a lot to prepare my body for healing, so when a treatment did become available, it would stand a better chance of working.

So I set about doing everything I could to create the conditions for healing in my body. My wellness plan included good nutrition, vitamins, laughter, meditation, visualization, prayer, regular exercise, educating myself, and doing volunteer work at a local AIDS organization. Making survival a full-time job didn't give me time to sit around feeling depressed.

With the help of caring friends and health care providers, I soon discovered that I could still dance! I could still laugh! I could still enjoy my friends and my life. I could still be joyfully alive, even with AIDS and cancer.

I have found there is hope even in facing death. When I was close to death from AIDS complications, I was amazed at how my hope and faith gave me courage. Sometimes hope in the face of death comes from what a person believes about life after death; sometimes it is simply the expectation of release from pain and suffering.

Shortly after my "terminal" diagnosis, my therapist taught me the Native American saying, "The quality of life is not measured by the length of life, but by the fullness with which we enter each present moment." This, too, gave me hope: I learned to live in the moment, and to use each moment to improve my chances of survival.

Living and dying with HIV/AIDS can be an experience of loneliness and despair. I know that experience can be transformed into a life of hope, through empowering those of us living with HIV/AIDS to be actively alive until we die. This creates hope, even when life seems hopeless. What greater gift can a caregiver offer?

— Reverend A. Stephen Pieters

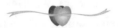

The Care and Feeding of Caregivers

How can you tell if someone is a caregiver? Well, he or she is probably sleepy! That's because the job description may include being available day and night, and after a while, it's hard to tell which is which. If you are a caregiver for a person with Parkinson's Disease (PWP), you soon discover that sleep irregularities and insomnia are part of the package for many PWPs. In addition, nighttime medications and journeys to the bathroom are customary in the later stages of this so-called designer disease.

We call it that because no two PWP's experience the disease in quite the same way. The progression of symptoms, even which ones are present, varies from person to person. And, of course, that means the medications, the schedule on which they are taken, and the reactions to them also vary.

For example, most people think of tremor as the major symptom of Parkinson's. Many, my husband among them, have little or no tremor but do exhibit the other major symptoms of rigidity and slowness (bradykinesia), as well as depression, tiny handwriting, gastrointestinal problems, and swallowing, to name a few. The list covers them literally from head to toe.

This presents the caregivers, and the loved ones we care for, with a baffling array of issues to contend with. As the disease progresses, and medications become less effective, we have to keep up with the latest developments, carefully track our PWP's progress, be sure the neurologist is informed of changes, decide what assistive aids are needed for daily living, and, of course, manage somehow to take care of ourselves.

Some of us are blessed with supportive friends and family and live in communities where there are resources that offer excellent care for our PWPs. Others may be isolated, socially or geographically, and may not have the understanding support of other family members or the financial resources to hire help when the care of our PWP becomes more than we can manage alone. In some cases, the fact that we live at a distance from the PWP makes it hard to know what is really going on, or to find appropriate help at the other end.

This job is not one we applied for—or, in most cases, ever expected to have. We're learning on the job, and need all the help we can get! The journey of Parkinson's disease was not one chosen, but our loved ones are on that journey, and we must accompany them. Therefore, I think of caregiving as accompaniment.

The accompanist at a concert is not the one you focus on, and that happens with caregivers, too. A well-meaning friend will ask, "How's John?" but seldom is the first question, "How are you?"

In a deeper sense, to accompany means to go, stay, or be connected with another person, to support that person not only physically, but emotionally and even spiritually as well. In this sense, caregivers are truly accompanists— whether on a daily, hands-on basis or from a distance.

A word about my personal experience is appropriate here. In addition to being a full-time caregiver for my husband, I am the founder and facilitator of an Internet discussion list for caregivers of PWPs. A sublist of a larger Parkinson list, the CARE list (which stands for Caregiver's Are Really Essential) has some 350 members in seventeen countries. I am privileged to share in their lives, to learn of their joys and frustrations.

I'd like to tell you a little about some of the things I've learned from them in the past three years on CARE. Most important is that caregivers need to know they are not alone, even if they are isolated by the demands of caregiving. There may be no local support group, and doctors may be too busy to listen and answer questions. Thus, the Internet may be their only contact with others who share their problems. And, it can offer support of all kinds—practical advice such as how to deal with home health agencies, how to tell a spouse he or she can't drive any more; emotional support when one has to helplessly watch a loved one suffer, or when relatives offer criticism rather than assistance.

Here is an excerpt from a message sent to CARE by a member in India. He wrote: "One of the nicest things for a caregiver is a little audience ... an opportunity to let off some steam, and [have] a platform for sharing. I think CARE is one of the best things that happened to me. I now feel part of a family that can actually respond with words of advice and encouragement ... something that's hard to find in today's fast-paced world ... thanks once again, I feel much better already!"

Another caregiver wrote, "I don't know if I'm looking for advice or just want to sound off ... but I am really at my wit's end and wondering if others are dealing with the same problems and if there are any viable solutions." She immediately received about a dozen replies, ranging from shared experiences with similar problems to encouragement and support in hiring help in a situation she could no longer manage alone.

Then there were the caregivers who wrote, "I'm not allowed to be sick. I have to be there for him," or "This disease changes the whole family—we've all lost control of our lives," or "Our plans for the future just went down the drain," or "I feel so guilty that I'm not a good enough caregiver, because I lose my temper a lot, and I should be comforting her."

Saddest of all are the words of the husband who wrote of his wife, "I'm losing her a little at a time, and it's so hard."

All these comments tell of what I call stress by association, for just as we know that any kind of stress can aggravate the symptoms of Parkinson's, we know it also makes caregiving harder. Here's where the support of family and friends can help so much—by focusing on the accompanist and on what it takes to help him or her make that unasked-for journey as a companion to the PWP.

The Internet offers a wide range of resources for caregivers, but not all of us are Net surfers, so it is important to learn some other ways to relieve stress and preserve your sanity as a caregiver. You may have developed your own coping mechanisms that work reliably and well for you. If not, consider some of these:

- Keep a journal of your feelings, as a substitute for being able to talk with someone who understands, or talking to family members or friends who are good listeners.
- Write poetry to distill the experiences you are having.
- Bang cupboard doors.
- Exercise, take a walk.
- Treat yourself to a favorite food (but be careful with this one).
- Learn all you can about the disease, to feel more prepared for the future.
- Focus on the present and the needs and rewards of the day.
- Seek the support of the faith community to which you belong.

There is, of course, a brighter side to caregiving: the satisfaction of being needed and being able to help someone you love. A good relationship becomes even deeper and more rewarding. You can test yourself and find that you are stronger and more capable than you ever dreamed . . . and that love and a sense of humor are the best coping mechanisms of all!

— Camilla Hewson Flintermann

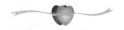

Breast Cancer—The Male Caregiver's Perspective

Your wife has just been diagnosed with breast cancer. Welcome to one of the hardest experiences the two of you will ever go through. Nothing can truly prepare you for this. But if you and your wife face this with the right attitude, it can become (as incredible as this may sound) one of the most rewarding experiences you will ever share.

When your spouse is diagnosed with breast cancer, your life is going to change. Some husbands choose to gloss over their wife's problem. Other husbands jump right in and take an active part in the decision-making and healing processes. Finally, some husbands are a combination of both. They may leave the decision about the treatment up to the wives, but they are there to provide emotional support.

When I first heard that my wife had cancer, it was as if I could not inhale. The news was devastating beyond comprehension. The first thing that crossed my mind was whether I would still have my best friend in a year, or would she become another depressing statistic? After a few hours, I was able to snap back to reality and begin to help my wife face her fears.

Because of the type of cancer and the size of the mass, she was scheduled for a modified radical mastectomy in two days. We did not have time to get a second opinion, but we were able to ask some other oncologists questions about what was going on and felt somewhat comfortable with our decision.

If you and your wife do not feel comfortable for any reason with a doctor's diagnosis or prescribed treatment, however, definitely seek another opinion and ask as many questions as you deem necessary. There is no such thing as a stupid question when it comes to the health of a loved one.

After the surgery is over and the healing begins, you may be more overwhelmed than you ever could have imagined. You will need to be there to help your wife do things she can no longer do alone, things that were so simple for her before.

If you have the joy of having children, as we do, your work never seems to end. Combine this with still having to go to your regular job, and you will soon find there is no time in the day for you.

When this cycle continues for an extended period of time, you can reach the edge of an emotional cliff. You may suffer emotional exhaustion or, as the professionals call it, caregiver burnout.

What seems to make things worse is that people constantly ask in-depth questions about how your wife is doing. Few, if any, however, ask how you are doing. When people did ask me, I almost felt selfish or complaining when I told the truth.

Don't feel you are being selfish. When people ask, be honest. Being honest helps to cleanse the emotions that have built up inside—fear, anger, resentment, sadness, or anything. Each person deals with this situation in a different manner. Letting someone else know how you feel helps them to understand why you are acting the way you are. Ignoring your emotions will only cause problems. Let them out and deal with them. This will not make you less of a man. Instead, it will make you more of a stable man.

In the beginning, you may find that you sacrifice most of yourself to establish a caregiving routine. But after the routine is set, try to take some time for yourself. You need to do this to keep your sanity while in the midst of things over which you have no control.

Try to do something for yourself every day. It does not need to be planned, expensive, or lengthy. Take an extra ten minutes getting to work in the morning and listen to your favorite tape or take the scenic way home. If friends, neighbors, or family are helping, take time to treat yourself to something you have not done in a long time. Whatever it is, do something just for yourself.

Caregiver burnout is not your wife's fault or anyone else's; it's just one of the side effects of healing. Realize that you are a very important part of the healing process, both physically and emotionally. If you are burned out or stressed out, you can't create a good healing environment.

Everyone wants to get through the ordeal as quickly and safely as possible. Recognizing in advance that you may feel added stress, and having some idea of how to deal with it, can help to improve the healing environment. You will have time to do things with your wife after the healing is done. In the meantime, don't forget yourself.

— Judd Lewis Parsons

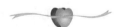

Migraine Headaches

There is no other pain quite like it, and you—or your care recipient—won't even know which bothers you more, the throbbing, vomiting, nausea, or seeing spots. Symptoms of migraine headaches can be so excruciating that you find yourself or your loved one attempting unusual tactics just to get some relief, such as lying facedown on cold bathroom tile. It may provide a temporary break from migraine symptoms, but as soon as you attempt to become active, the pain comes shooting right back. Migraines can last for days or weeks, disrupting your job, family life, or social life.

More than twenty-eight million Americans suffer from recurring migraine headaches, and 70 percent of them are women. Unfortunately, more than half of migraine sufferers go undiagnosed by a physician, according to the National Headache Foundation (NHF). It is unclear why migraine pain is triggered, but 145 million workdays are lost annually because of it. Factors that contribute to the onset of a migraine include fatigue, bright lights, hormones, stress, and certain foods.

With the growing number of people living with migraine pain, primary doctors are becoming increasingly more informed about migraine headaches and the treatment options available. As a patient or caregiver, you can establish better communication with your health care provider to find a successful treatment program for yourself or your loved one. The NHF has released ten specific steps to communicate better with health care providers:

- **Seek help.** Be a self-advocate. There is no need for you or your care recipient to suffer with migraine pain when new treatment options are available. Seek out information about migraine headaches so you can communicate more effectively with your doctor.

- **Educate yourself about migraines so you will know what to communicate to a physician.** A variety of sources provide information about migraine pain on the Web, including the NHF at www.headaches.org or call (800) NHF-5552.

- **Make a doctor's appointment to discuss your or your loved one's headaches.** Find out if you or your care recipient's primary doctor knows about migraine headaches and treatments. If not, you may want to seek out a headache specialist or neurologist.

- **Prepare for a dialogue with your physician.** Keep a headache diary. Be ready to tell the physician when migraine headaches occur, how long they last, what precedes migraine onset, symptoms, and severity of pain. Note any missed workdays or social engagements due to migraine pain. If medication is prescribed, track its effectiveness at pain relief and how long that relief lasts.

- **Have realistic expectations about treatment.** There is no cure for migraines, but managing them is possible. When working with a physician, stay open-minded about trying new treatments. Treatment success could ebb and flow, so prepare to modify it.

- **Be honest with the physician about all medications taken or any medical condition.** To prevent adverse drug reactions, inform the doctor about all prescribed or over-the-counter medications.

- **Stay optimistic about the treatment.** Don't give up. Instead, focus on collaborating with the doctor to find a solution, even though it may take time.

- **Read and ask the doctor for detailed instructions about all medication that has been prescribed.** All prescription medication comes with instructions:

when to take it, how much to take, if it should be taken with water or food, etc. Ask the physician about anything you don't understand.

- **Form a partnership with the physician concerning treatment success.** Treatment has a greater chance of success with regular visits with the physician and open communication lines.

- **Follow up regularly with the doctor.** The effectiveness of treatment depends on the time invested and follow-up visits. Make the next appointment before leaving the office. (Physicians usually recommend three months between visits.)

— National Headache Foundation, *Today's Caregiver Magazine*

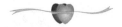

Colon Cancer Care List

When the diagnosis is colon cancer, what are your responsibilities as a caregiver? Here is a quick list:

- Call your local county medical association to find a physician with significant experience with the type of cancer diagnosed.

- Get a second opinion (but not a fourth or fifth) from someone of equal or better ability and qualifications than your physician.

- Insist on adequate and appropriate pain management.

- Investigate complementary therapies as a supplement to the physician's care, not as a replacement.

- Maintain a high-fiber/low-carbohydrate diet. Consult a nutritionist and don't force your loved one to eat.

- Make and keep appointments. Recurrences can happen without warning, so the only way to catch colon cancer while it can still be treated is to maintain a regular schedule of checkups, including a colonoscopy.

- After diagnosis, encourage your loved one to keep healthy routines as much as possible and do normal tasks, even going back to work (if permitted) as soon as possible.

- Your loved one may feel anger or denial, become sullen, or develop an altered sense of self-worth, body image, and sexuality. Reassure him or her that your feelings have not changed, and provide the emotional support your loved one needs by listening and talking with him or her honestly.

- Find and attend cancer support groups for both of you.

— Today's Caregiver Magazine

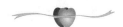

Surviving the Caregiver's Role

On June 10, 1990, our lives were turned upside down. Our fifteen-year-old daughter, Terri-Lynn, was out joyriding with friends when the car rolled, and she was thrown 140 feet. She suffered a severe massive brain injury. Her improvement has been extremely slow but is ongoing. She still cannot be left alone at all and requires twenty-four-hour-a-day care.

I am still here, after eight years, and I can laugh and cry and make responsible decisions. I have learned that every patient is different, and that every caregiver comes to the role with a different background. Each person has to find his or her own way of being a caregiver, but I would like to share some of the things that have helped me survive in this role.

Finding a Counselor

Finding a counselor who could help me learn to recognize and face my feelings of frustration and anger, while learning to let myself grieve, was an immense help. Caregivers often fall into the trap of beating ourselves up over feelings we are not comfortable with. It is so important to stop judging ourselves: there are plenty of other people doing that for us.

Sense of Humor

It seems impossible during the initial stages of trauma, but somewhere under all the stress is our sense of humor. Finding that humor was sometimes the only thing that I felt kept me sane and able to handle impossible situations.

Basic Instincts

As a parent, it is very difficult to realize that caring for your child is part of someone's job, so the people taking care of him or her are not emotionally involved. They go home after their shift and live their own lives. It is also difficult for them to remember, at times, that this child is part of you, and not just your job, and this is your life. I had to learn to follow my instincts and not worry about what the professionals thought. The rehabilitation department stopped Terri-Lynn's rehabilitation therapy after two years, because she was not going to improve. But I continued to work on it. I had to ignore their comments about wasting my time and go on with what I felt was necessary. Now, Terri-Lynn plays computer games and volunteers, playing cards with children in a day care center. I know it was right to follow my heart. Parents can't close the chart and go home after eight hours.

Support Groups

There are support groups in a lot of cities and on the Internet. Talking to people who are also caregivers and who understand just how tiring or frustrating life can be has been a tremendous help. A chat room is an excellent place to vent some of these feelings and listen to others vent as well. It has the advantage of being anonymous, and most of us have found it so much easier to talk to people we don't see every day, but who understand. The other advantage to a chat room is that the other people are there at 10 P.M., when I get a chance to take a break. I don't have to get a respite worker in to be able to spend time with these friends. Noncaregivers would be very surprised to hear just how much laughing and real stress release happens in a chat room.

There are always lots of people who have no experience with what I am living with, who think they know what I should do, or what they would do if they were me. It took me a long time to learn to remember that they aren't me, and they aren't in my position, and, therefore, they have no idea what they would do. I realize they mean well, but I resent their thinking they could run my life better than I can. I have had to learn to think of these people as the old aunt who never had kids, but was an authority on how to raise them. This is where a sense of humor is most required.

Asking for Help

You know best how people can help you out. Learning to ask for help was another sanity-saving act. I found a couple of friends who were glad to help out once they knew what they could do. I asked them to sit here for an hour and let me go shopping, or let my husband and me go out for supper. These are all simple, basic things that seem to take a while to occur to a caregiver. Learning to speak up and ask for help for yourself is as necessary as speaking up and acting as an advocate for the person you are caring for. Often, caregivers believe themselves to be irreplaceable. Reminding myself that cemeteries are full of irreplaceable people has helped at times. I can't take care of my daughter if I don't take care of (and take time for) my own needs.

Hired Help

Another part of taking care of myself was hiring someone for a few hours a week to come in and spend time with Terri-Lynn. The rates for respite workers vary, and not everyone can afford them, but I found a wonderful solution for anyone who has a nursing school nearby. Student nurses are cheaper to hire for someone who doesn't need actual nursing care, and they are glad to have the experience of working one-on-one with people. It also gives them practical experience to list on their resumes. Interview and hire a couple of them, so you always have a backup. As a caregiver, you suddenly realize that life has gone on for your friends, and you are out of touch with them. We have learned to phone and invite people over because they never know when I am busy with Terri-Lynn and don't stop in the way they used to.

Solitude

Praying for strength and finding some quiet time alone—even for half an hour—is also something that has helped me regroup and refresh. When I calm down, I can tell people who think I should get on with my life that this is my life, and I am getting on with it the best way I can.

— Carol Nahls

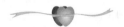

Surviving a Fractured Hip

Fractured hips are a leading cause of disability. Such fractures usually require surgery, leaving your loved one somewhat incapacitated. Among the deficits experienced, your loved one will temporarily lose the ability to bend forward, twist his or her body, or pick a leg up off the bed. These deficits will be compounded by a lack of endurance.

As a result, additional demands are placed on the caregiver. Recovery can take up to nine months. Some preparation before a loved one comes home from the hospital will reduce the demands on the caregiver and facilitate recovery.

Prepare by making a few purchases and modifying the home slightly. The caregiver should purchase:

- **A reacher** to help your loved one pick up items from the floor or those just out of reach, and put on pants or underwear.

- **A long shoehorn** so the patient can put on his or her shoes without bending forward.

- **Shoes that do not tie.** Either loafers or tennis shoes with Velcro closures are better. For ladies, a simple slip-on style without heels is another option.

- **A long-handled bath sponge** so your loved one can wash his or her legs without bending forward.

- **A bath seat with a back for the bathtub or shower stall.** Sitting while showering will conserve your loved one's energy and eliminate the possibility of a fall while bathing.

- **A handheld showerhead.** Sitting in a shower with a fixed head gives the sensation of being in a waterfall. Having a handheld showerhead gives your loved one control over the direction of the water flow.

Most of these items can be found in local department or specialty stores, with the exception of the reacher, which can be purchased through an outpatient clinic with therapy services. Comparison shopping is strongly recommended for the bath seat, as prices can vary greatly. Features to consider are rubber tips on all four legs to keep the seat from sliding, anodized aluminum construction to prevent rust, and adjustable legs to raise or lower the seat height.

With regard to the home, the caregiver should:

- Remove all scatter and throw rugs. Walking will not be easy following surgery, and your loved one could trip on one of these.

- Move all electrical cords out of pathways in the home. Again, these are a hazard that could cause a fall.

- Provide a cordless telephone, if possible. This will allow your loved one some independence and communication with the outside world in case of an emergency.

- Provide a chair with armrests, which give support when moving to a standard position. The chair should *not* swivel or rock, because this could throw your loved one's balance off, and cause him or her to fall.

These general recommendations will help your loved one recover more quickly and safely, but he or she may continue to need more intensive therapy. The surgeon will be able to direct you more appropriately.

— L. Theresa Pantanella, O.T.R.

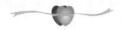

Coping Skills

The day you discover your child has cancer, your whole life changes. No matter what the outcome may be, you are now living on an emotional roller coaster. When my son was first diagnosed, he was scared and angry and embarrassed about losing his hair. The fact remained that, although he was now a cancer patient, he was still a fourteen-year-old with all the typical emotions, feelings, and concerns of that age. For me, being a single mother and becoming a caregiver at the same time meant I had to find new skills to cope with this dreadful disease. I have included some of them here.

Trust

Choose a doctor who is not only qualified, but one who is able to speak comfortably with you and your child. Make sure the doctor takes the time to answer your questions and those of your child.

Communication

Be open and honest with your child and, as much as possible, include him or her in discussions about treatment. Listen with your heart.

Understanding

Know that your child may take out most of his or her anger on you. After all, you are the one who will continue to love your child, no matter what. Be firm, but loving.

Support

Find a support group for parents where you can discuss your fears and concerns. It is very hard for family and friends to really understand what you are going through. Talk to the psychologist at the hospital and vent your anger.

Knowledge

You will be asked to make many decisions during the course of treatment. Read and learn as much as you can about your child's illness. The more you understand, the better prepared you will be to cope.

Humor

As hard as it may seem, keep your sense of humor. Do fun things with your child and laugh. Remember, your child stills wants to be treated as the person you knew before he or she became ill.

Friends and Family

Don't expect others to know how to react or what to say. Be specific when asking them for support: baby-sitting, car-pooling, a cooked meal, etc.

Siblings

Remember, siblings' lives have changed too. They are also scared, and they may resent the lack of attention. Do spend quality time with them and listen to their fears. An excellent organization, Candlelighters Childhood Cancer Foundation, puts out a quarterly newsletter as well as a youth newsletter that encourages kids to tell their stories and seek pen pals. For more information, or to request a free subscription, call (800) 366-2223. Chai Lifeline is another organization that gives support to families with children who have a life-threatening disease. It can be reached at (212) 255-1160 or (305) 956-9990. Although my son did not survive his battle with cancer, I hope, through my experience, to help other parents cope with being a caregiver.

— Sandi Magadov

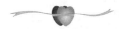

Helping Children Deal with Loss

Today, more and more American families are involved in the care of their loved ones. Often this changes family dynamics, altering routines, roles, economic status, stress levels, and demands on adult time for all of the family members involved. The changes taking place create loss and loss creates grief. A grieving child needs our reassurance that he or she is loved and will be cared for.

It is extremely important to listen to your children verbalize their fears, anger, confusion, and doubts. We should explain that grief and the feelings it evokes are natural responses to loss. We must encourage our children to express their sadness by sharing their thoughts, feelings, and memories with trusted listeners.

Illness can be sudden or it can creep into our loved one's life in stages, as in Alzheimer's disease. Our loved one may be dealing with the loss of health, independence, and, in some cases, ultimately the loss of life. The family deals with these losses as well.

The changes associated with the disease are threatening for our loved one, our children, and ourselves. It is important to take the time to discuss the disease with children so they can understand what is happening to their loved one.

Children and teens may experience a wide range of emotions. All too often, caregivers are too overwhelmed by their own shock, sadness, and grief to notice that their children are grieving too. For children, as adults, there is no magic wand to overcome grief. It is a process as individual as the people going through it.

The stages of grief are not linear. There will be ups and downs, peaks and valleys, and the inevitable bumps in the road. Shock, denial, anger, regression, guilt, bargaining, and, finally, acceptance are the myriad emotions that are part of the healing process called grief.

For some children, keeping a journal is a wonderful way to facilitate the grieving process. Encourage them to draw their feelings; I call this type of drawing *heart art.* Young children think symbolically rather than in words: pictures reveal their thinking. Drawing actually helps children find their words. Journal exercises can offer insights into a child's fears and misconceptions. Keeping a journal allows children to express themselves creatively. Use their drawings as a springboard for caring conversations. For older children and teens, writing in a journal gives them permission to record their feelings and emotions. It allows them to feel close to their loved one and remember happier times, and it provides an opportunity to say good-bye. This is a very important step toward acceptance in the grieving process.

Remember, children are experiencing life just as you are; they are not just in a getting ready phase. Because disease and death are part of those real-life experiences, they inevitably will touch your children and your family in some way. Coping with the loss of a loved one is one of the most difficult challenges adults and children will ever face. To understand the grieving process and to be guided through the stages of grief by the loving, gentle hands of a caring, compassionate adult empowers children. We are teaching our children important coping skills that will serve them well the rest of their lives.

— Katherine Dorn Zotovich

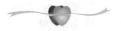

Ask Dr. Ghen

Q: I have read a lot about alternative treatments for cancer. How do I know which ones will be helpful for my relative's cancer?—P.R., Rhode Island

Don't believe for one second that any or all of these so-called treatments are cures for cancer. Cancer represents more than a hundred distinct different diseases. A single treatment for cancer would be like prescribing the same topical antibiotic for a cut or a cough.

Seek a trained professional alternative physician who has gained a good knowledge of many different modalities that may be helpful in the treatment of a particular cancer. Do not let wild claims of 100 percent success, 100 percent cures, or the like, make you buy these products. You may just be disappointed and poorer when you are finished.

Stay away from any product that claims that its ingredients are a secret. Again, find the individual who can give you a well-rounded, intelligent, focused, and integrated treatment plan.

Q: I have chronic fatigue syndrome. What can I do about it?—I.R., Florida

Unfortunately, chronic fatigue syndrome (CFS) probably has many etiologies. We used to believe that it was related just to the Epstein-Barr virus; however, we now think there are many probable causes. Do not despair; it is important to treat this like any chronic disease and look for the underlying reasons for your continued fatigue. Areas your doctor will want to evaluate include:

- Epstein-Barr virus titers;
- general blood work for liver function, blood count, cholesterol, triglycerides, sodium, potassium, magnesium, B12, and folic acid;
- studies to evaluate the adrenal gland; and
- testing for heavy metal toxicity, including mercury, cadmium, aluminum, lead, arsenic, antimony, and platinum.

Treatment should be directed toward improvement of cellular nutrition, which means prescribing appropriate individualized vitamins, minerals, amino acids, and possibly even herbals. I have found from my clinical experience that patients with this syndrome often require several intravenous vitamin and mineral infusions to improve the severe cellular depletion of these nutrients.

One of the difficult problems often presenting with this syndrome is significant depression. Make certain your health care practitioner addresses this issue with conventional antidepressants or nutraceuticals or both.

Most important, emotional support is required from families and friends. If you are a caregiver, realize that patients with CFS often experience exhaustion as debilitating as the most severe of chronic diseases. With an appropriate workup and good nutritional support, along with the appropriate medicine, you should expect positive results. Try keeping positive thoughts in your mind and keep dancing (exercise)!

Q: I am taking care of somebody who has AIDS. Are there any natural remedies to boost her immune system? — P.H., Oregon

It is very important for people with AIDS to maintain good nutrition. Remove those items from the diet that reduce T cell function and compromise the overall immune status. Sugars, white flours, and fried foods should be avoided. Consider getting a juicer or Vitamix that pulverizes and liquefies whole foods, making fruits and vegetables the main staple in the diet. If possible buy organically grown fruits and vegetables; if that is not possible, rinse and wash the foods either with 3 percent food-grade hydrogen peroxide for ten minutes or use castille soap, such as the one made by Dr. Bronner's. Both will remove most of the pesticides and other residues.

Exercise is also extremely important for people with compromised immune systems; however, too much or too little exercise can reduce the white blood cell count. I suggest a combination of light weight lifting and aerobic exercise five days a week for twenty to thirty minutes at a time. Also, I suggest adding 1,000 mg of L-glutamine in a powdered form to a glass of water and drinking it after each exercise period. This amino acid gets used up quickly during vigorous exercise, and it plays an integral part in maintaining the immune system. Stretching, such as yoga and tai chi, is also wonderful for toning the body.

Check laboratory data for DHEA (dehydroepiandrosterone) levels and somatomedin-C and restore these hormones, if deficient, to the normal ranges. See if you can find a physician who can examine the patient's blood, saliva, and urine for biological terrain, a specialized study that may help determine whether the body's environment is in its optimal state.

Vitamin and mineral replacement should be individualized, but certain vitamins and minerals are imperative for good health of the HIV/AIDS patient, particularly antioxidants; A, C, and E; beta-carotene; selenium; and glutathione.

State of mind is extremely important as well and can positively or adversely affect the immune function. Many studies have shown that the proper attitude and state of mind can significantly improve T cell activity function and overall T cell total. Whatever process brings the patient to an altered state of consciousness and a feeling of wellness should be incorporated into the total treatment regime. Some examples of techniques that are quite helpful are neurolinguistic programming, meditation, prayer, and guided imagery.

Try to develop a relationship with a physician well versed in natural immune support so the patient does not try to take everything at one time. Using a scientific approach to alternatives, and applying those various modalities and supplements that are most beneficial to an HIV/AIDS patient, will yield better results than indiscriminate combinations of these substances.

— Mitchell Ghen, D.O., Ph.D.

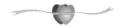

Best of Health

I supervise students in local acupuncture school clinics. One lesson for my students is how to feel compassion while not absorbing the energies of their patients. Often my students think they can best serve their patients by somehow identifying with them and even taking on their pain and suffering. Students usually discuss the case with me before I see the patient, and often I have had students act out their patient's physical characteristics and mental attitude. It's as if the students feel the more they can take in the suffering of the patients, the better that they will be at healing them.

Then there are patients who aren't satisfied until the doctor feels as bad as they do. Obviously, these are patients with boundary problems, as are the doctors who have to take on the patient's pain as their own. In both cases, the patient and doctor are in a *co-dependent* relationship.

This is an important issue for caregivers. Often the things that affect us most are those we most identify with. Being afraid of your own illness and death is obviously an impediment to being able to see the suffering of others compassionately. Your denial can be transmitted to the patient.

This is much, much harder when we deal with a family member. I have special compassion for those whose family members are ill or have passed on. Your parent or sibling or child is a genetic part of you. This is not an "other" person; this is someone with your own DNA code and, as such, facing the ill health or death of a parent is irrefutable proof of your own mortality. I make it clear to people in this situation that there are no harder times than these. When a relative is ill, there is often nothing to do but experience the grief. It is not a time to try to rationalize or analyze complex emotions.

Healers (and caregivers) call on their own spiritual beliefs to witness the pain of others, while not absorbing them. Nowhere is this territory explored more than in writings by Stephen Levine, Ondrea Levine, and Ram Dass (Richard Alpert). *In Healing into Life and Death,* Stephen Levine writes,

> You are reacting to their world, not responding to yours. Indeed, their reactions have nothing to do with you. Emotions are not rational, nor need they be. To attempt to make them rational is to cause great conflict within. But to simply watch how the mind emotes, how it smiles and frowns in reaction to the world, can give some insight into its natural unfoldings. When the world is allowed within the heart, we deeply understand there is nothing to judge and all our healings are based on intention.

— Douglas Eisenstark, L.Ac.

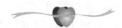

Natural Alternatives for Insomnia

I was reading a newspaper article the other day about insomnia and the symptoms that generally accompany lack of sleep. It was interesting to note that neither preventive nor alternative approaches were mentioned, despite the fact that nearly 47 percent of the population suffers from one form or another, and a number of proven treatments are available.

Several different types of insomnia come to mind, but the most obvious definition is the inability to maintain regular sleep patterns on a consistent basis for more than three weeks. One of the major causes of insomnia is a malfunction of the pituitary and its inability to manufacture sufficient levels of serotonin.

How can insomnia be prevented? Not easily. But on further consideration, alternatives to the traditional medical approach may provide more than adequate solutions. By focusing on the person as an individual and searching for specific symptoms and clues associated with causes, explanations become a bit easier. Once the underlying causes are eliminated, balance, health, and, more important, sleep, are recovered.

In looking at any type of physical or emotional imbalance, one of the first places to start is the bowel. Questioning what the bowel has to do with sleep, we begin where everything ends. The intestinal track comprises almost 40 percent of the immune system. When it is out of balance, the remainder of the system cannot function properly. Toxins, parasites, candida, and bacteria (some friendly and some not) live in the intestine. Daily elimination and a clean bowel create an environment where disease cannot thrive.

The strange part is that we often take better care of our cars or clothes than we do our bowel. A company called ReNew Life has an easy-to-use product for bowel cleansing that is carried in most health food stores. Follow the label and eat whole foods as much as possible.

Many companies offer colon cleansers, and if you have found one that is effective for you, use it, but not all the time. Infrequent use allows the bowel to reestablish its own natural tendencies, which is the ultimate purpose of these products.

We hear the terms *cleanse* and *detoxify* more frequently than we might like. When it comes to bodily functions, each is interpreted differently. We detoxify the organs and glands, then cleanse the toxins from our system. This is the next step in prevention: detoxifying the kidneys, liver, lungs, and skin. On occasion, a simple cleanse, after detoxification, is effective.

The steps necessary to complete a detoxification and cleanse are another article in themselves. Several companies, including Eden's Secret, Solaray's Total Cleanse, ReNew Life, Gaia Herbs, manufacture detox and cleanse programs. See which ones fit your lifestyle, and include fresh fruit and vegetables for a few weeks to assist in the process. Also, add more good protein to allow the liver to eliminate poisons from your system.

Consider eliminating the following, at least during the detoxification and cleansing period. If absolutely necessary, add them back in one at a time to determine if they may have been the cause of insomnia: coffee, cigarettes, soda, artificial sweeteners, processed foods, processed wheat products, soy, canola, sugar, milk and dairy (including ice cream), and meat products. The exact reasons for each has to do with its effect on the bowel, liver, and pituitary.

Antioxidant formulas are essential in reestablishing the immune system and are also helpful in the cleansing process, along with protein powders, such as whey, rice, or vegetable. Protein powders help the liver eliminate toxins, as mentioned above. Some antioxidants to consider: alpha-lipoic acid, N-acetyl cysteine, green tea, beta-carotene (mixed carotenoid), vitamin E (mixed tocopherol), vitamin C, selenium, methyl sulfonyl methane, garlic, and rosemary.

With stronger physical, mental, and emotional health, sleep may improve naturally. If not, some additional preventive techniques may help:

- **Maintain a healthy lifestyle:** This includes diet, exercise, elimination or reduction of chemicals and nutrient-poor foods, and a prevention attitude.

- **Reduce stress and anxiety:** Find a calming method that works for your temperament (meditation tapes, deep-breathing exercises, yoga, creative activities, visualization, etc.).

- **Take vitamins and supplements:** Look for a daily regime that's not overwhelming and stick to it. Necessities include a multivitamin, a multimineral, enzymes, a fatty acid complex, and amino acids.

- **Evaluate your sleep habits:** Is the room dark enough? Are there noises? Have you considered using "white" noises? Is the mattress comfortable? Are there digital clocks or TVs near the bed? Do you use a water bed with a heating element? These are all important questions whose answers may require adjusting your sleep environment.

- **Eliminate suppressed emotions:** Physical and emotional chaos can come from unexpressed emotions. Find a healthy release. Discuss your problems and communicate your needs. Screaming only creates more stress on the adrenals and the heart, so use a more constructive approach. Try writing about your feelings in a journal if communication or discussion is impossible.

- **Try a hot bath or shower.**

The idea is not only to find a ritual that calms and relaxes, but one that is easy to maintain and continue. I have a patient who lies on his back, crosses one foot over the other, and contemplates the best parts of his day, while breathing deeply. Eventually, he is able to turn onto his side and sleep.

As a society, we generally tend to follow traditional approaches and ingest medications that may mask underlying symptoms or create undesirable side effects. In comparison, most of the alternative approaches mentioned here are safe, inexpensive, and nontoxic.

One of the major concerns of alternative and traditional health practitioners is self-prescribing. I recommend finding a health care practitioner who can assist in your evaluation while guiding your choices.

Sleep problems and their side effects are far too important to neglect. Better sleep provides better health and well-being.

— David Dancu, N.D., J.D.

Chapter 7

Depression, Guilt, and Fear

Alzheimer's

There's been changes lately, ma
A monster's taking you
This time the enemy is within

Who you are is sinking
Sinking with your glance
It's your daughters' eyes

Our hands are clasped around you
As our center fades away

We held them to the wall
Until the monster had a name
No Not her Not this
She's battled governments

Just once more ma stand
Stand and fight Goddamn it fight

And now that you've surrendered
Be comforted Be sure
Along this final front
Four brave soldiers in hushed alarm
Will march with you

— © Pamela R. Clayton

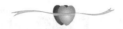

When Guilt Comes Knocking

Guilt—isn't that a familiar word? You would think that mature rational adults like us would be above feeling guilt about the emotions our caregiving can evoke. Not so. I am a mature and rational adult. I am a registered nurse who works with the elderly and their families. I counseled these same families on how to deal with everyday issues, including guilt.

Yet, there I was, reduced at times to a quivering mass of jelly by a word or a look from my parents. I took care of my parents for more than seventeen years. And, it took every bit of those seventeen years for me to realize how easily I reacted to the buttons my parents have pushed to get me to do what they wanted. It often caused untold hardship in my personal life, yet I refused to see it for what it was. Worse, I refused to take appropriate action to ensure that it did not happen again.

It was finally through the wonder of a truly magical medium—the Internet—that I was able to recognize and deal with guilt. There were days that I would rather not live through again, and there is still a little part of me that feels a twinge every now and then. But I survived the journey, and I am here to tell every one of you out there that there is help for you.

We help each other. We support each other. And we make caregiving a little easier for each other. The fact that you are here is one of the first steps in getting that help. I am no expert. But I am a caregiver who has had to deal with all sorts of problems.

Dealing with Guilt

Okay, enough of the clichés, you say. How *do* you deal with the guilt? I can give you a list of references, but I found that just reading about something doesn't always cut it for me. So I will try to express here one or two things that I found helpful.

Once I was able to recognize that I felt guilty, I had to realize as well that no one gave it to me. Guilt is a self-made emotion. We do it to ourselves. We take those words or actions of others and internalize them, probably because we are looking for a reason to be guilty. Whatever the reason for guilt, it is wasted energy. It is energy that we could be using for good, healthy, and productive activities.

Kate's Rule Number 1: Never Go to Sleep Feeling Guilty!

Really, I mean it! Each night before I go to sleep, before I ask God for strength to get through tomorrow, or thank Him for today's blessings, I ask myself one question: Do I believe in my heart that I have done the best that I could today for my loved one and myself? Notice I said *myself.* If I fail to do the best for myself, how can I possibly be any good to anyone else? And never mind what others have to say about what you are doing or how you are doing it. *You* are the one providing care, and *you* are the one living it every day. What you believe about your actions is all that matters. And if I truly believe that I have done my best on this one day, then I have absolutely nothing to feel guilty about.

So the next time guilt comes knocking at your door, don't answer. Leave it outside where it belongs. And when you put your head down on that pillow tonight, rest easy knowing that you are doing the very best that you can with what you have been given.

— Catherine Murphy, R.N.

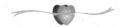

Signs of Depression

It's often difficult to differentiate between sadness and depression. Each has certain qualities that frequently overlap, yet both can affect our lives dramatically. Sadness can range from simple, momentary unhappiness to long-term grief or sorrow. Depression is defined as gloominess or dejection, either of which can be debilitating. With the realization or diagnosis of either sadness or depression, there is a tendency for physicians to quickly prescribe anti-depressant medication to mask and suppress negative feelings. I wouldn't say this is necessarily a good thing, because failing to address the true cause only prolongs rather than alleviates the problem.

Fortunately, there are alternatives to consider, such as mild exercise and more light. One can take a walk in the evening after dinner during the longer days of summer. In the winter months, better lighting in the house and walking around a mall or other large area help alleviate the lack of specific brain chemicals that may cause depression.

What are the typical symptoms of depression? How do you know whether depression is even an issue? There are four key areas to consider: behavior, appearance, feelings, and communication. With respect to behavior, we generally look for changes in so-called normal behavior patterns. A person may show disinterest in his or her usual surroundings or neglect to perform regular chores.

Symptoms of depression include:

- A change in usual behavior patterns
- A greater desire to be alone
- Sleeping more than usual
- Forgetfulness
- Loss of appetite

This isn't to say that other factors should not be considered, but given the following additional symptoms, depression is a primary diagnosis.

Appearance is something that is difficult to hide. As a caregiver, you should pay attention to uncombed hair, dirty clothes, facial expressions, unusual quietness, skin tone, and gestures. Concealing one's feelings may be easier for some than others, but obvious feelings may be more apparent. Look for recent signs of grief from the loss of a loved one or a pet or a sense of hopelessness with unusual anger and impatience. Also look for new or unusual reactions, such as self-blame or ongoing criticism of friends and relatives.

Finally, pay attention to the words being used. Some words and phrases are reflective of suicidal thoughts based on underlying depression. The key is to be aware of unusual behavior or words and take action before the person reaches a self-destructive or suicidal stage. These can include phrases like:

"I wish I were dead."

"What's the point of living?"

"I have no joy in my life."

"Things will be better when I'm gone."

"They won't have me to kick around much longer."

As a preliminary response, you might consider counseling. Please bear in mind that depression is difficult to self-diagnose, but the feeling that something is not right, with a chronic desire to sleep all the time, should lead one to consider help.

— David Dancu, J.D., N.D.

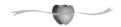

Depression in the Caregiver

Depression seems to be part and parcel of becoming a caregiver to a loved one. Depression is, in reality, anger turned inward. This is not always obvious, nor is it easily acknowledged. There are so many times we experience anger along the way as we watch our loved ones struggle to do simple tasks, watch them decline in mind and body, watch them lose their independence and, eventually, their lives in the process.

We, as caregivers, also experience many losses of our own simultaneously. We realize we are totally helpless in the face of encroaching illness and intense suffering. We cannot wave a magic wand and give our loved ones back their sense of control, nor can we retain the delusion that we have much control ourselves. We are merely outstretched hands to help our loved ones live as comfortably as possible in the time they have left.

Often, depression stems from extended stress or is situational in origin. This is due to the tremendous responsibilities that fall to us as the caregiver, to give 100 percent and go beyond that many times over, doing whatever is necessary to ensure quality care for our loved ones.

There is also clinical depression, from which I suffer, which is biochemical and hereditary and wreaks great havoc in its wake. Some days I find it hard to keep going on, keep doing, keep giving. However, during those times while I was caregiving, I realized that it was my efforts that enhanced the quality of my mother's remaining days. Without my help, her suffering would have been intolerable. So, while I was unable to escape my depression, I was still quite aware that my contribution made a difference to another person's quality of life—and this knowledge outweighed the influence of chronic depression. The love I carried for my mother enabled me to rise above my own disabling depression and do what helped her to live out her final days with as much peace as possible.

As a believer in a power greater than I, I gained strength to do what was necessary at the time. Having faith does not preclude experiencing depression. We are human beings and react to rapidly changing situations and traumatic events. All I know for sure is that my mother's final days were richer for having me as her caregiver, and I will never regret what was required of me. This was my gift to her for giving me my own life.

While depression may be my lifetime companion, it has not succeeded in overcoming the love I carry in my heart for my mother. Becoming a caregiver requires a commitment to essentially bear another's burden. I am grateful for every single day that I made the choice to do this. I know, without any doubt, that my life made a positive difference, and this knowledge makes it all worthwhile.

— © 2000 Dorothy Womack

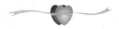

Anticipatory Grief

When we think of grief, we generally think of the process and feelings we experience after someone dies. In reality we begin this process on the day someone we love is diagnosed with a life-threatening illness. This process of mourning before someone we love has died is called *anticipatory grief*. According to noted grief expert Dr. Therese Rando, anticipatory grief refers to the process through which we begin to mourn past, present, and future losses.

Anticipatory grief is experienced by care recipients and caregivers from different perspectives. For instance, care recipients mourn the loss of their previous body image, changes in their physical and mental abilities, and, possibly, career loss. The role of the care recipient in the family may change. A breadwinner may no longer provide for the family, or a homemaker may no longer be able to manage the home independently.

Caregivers frequently take on these additional roles, while caring for their loved one and dealing with their own feelings. Both loved ones and caregivers are grieving for the way life was and the deterioration of the care recipient's health.

During the course of the illness there are many losses for the care recipient and primary caregiver. These may include intimacy, sex, privacy, independence, dreams, partnership, dignity, money, control, intellectual stimulation, friendship, and family position. These losses produce accompanying feelings of anger, sadness, depression, and abandonment. It is common for both the care recipient and caregiver to feel isolated, invisible, and numb. Frequently, the inability of friends and family members to manage their own discomfort with illness and death further isolates caregivers and their loved ones.

A long-term illness leaves a person with a mixed bag of feelings. As you watch someone you love in pain, you may wish that person to be out of his or her misery. This feeling can be followed by feelings of guilt and remorse, that we wished this person to die. Discussing these feelings is a survival necessity. Care recipients and caregivers need someone to hear and validate their feelings. Both parties require information about the illness, some support, and the means to maintain control over their lives, as they make the arduous journey toward death. Family members and close friends can be good sources of support, but if they are physically or emotionally unavailable, support groups and mental health professionals can be a greater source of support.

— Jennifer Kay, L.C.S.W.

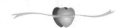

Exercising Away Depression

A survey by the National Ambulatory Care Association states that approximately seven million primary care visits are made annually for depression. Depressed individuals are also more apt to develop cardiovascular problems. Several studies have found that exercise and activity can help alleviate the symptoms of depression and improve the quality of life for individuals who suffer from depression. Though the exact reasons for exercise's positive impact on depression aren't clear, the findings are promising.

How Exercise May Help

Exercise may be an effective way to manage depression for several reasons.

- First, exercise that involves the use of large muscle groups may help relieve feelings of pent-up anxiety. Moving, stretching the muscles, the freedom of a full range of motion, and increasing circulation, for example, may help individuals release tension and aggression.

- Second, exercise improves one's physique, weight, and overall appearance. This can certainly help improve one's mood through enhanced self-esteem and confidence. Several of my clients have reported feeling less pressure because of their ability to eat more freely without gaining weight since they exercise.

- Being in control brings us to a third point. Individuals who exercise often feel better because they feel they are in control of themselves, their bodies, and, thus, their lives. A sense of mastery comes with the improved self-esteem exercise provides.

- Finally, exercise has been shown to produce beta-endorphins, the body's own morphine-like painkillers and source of euphoria. This "feel good" sensation is often referred to as runner's high.

How Much and How Often

Cardiovascular exercise can be defined as exercise that elevates the heart rate and sustains it for at least twenty minutes. If you can go thirty or forty minutes, that is even better, but start slowly. Running, biking, swimming, stair climbing, and even walking briskly are all ideal examples of cardiovascular activities. Aim to do such activity three times a week, or every other day. Cardiovascular exercise may improve not only your mood, but your weight, energy level, blood chemistry, and blood pressure as well.

When designing an exercise program for yourself or individuals with depression, a few additional factors need to be considered.

- Keep goals realistic. Set small, realistic, and measurable goals. Be sure to take baseline measurements of fitness before starting the program so you can chart progress.

- Weight, body fat percentage, body mass index (BMI), resting pulse rate, flexibility, circumferential measurements, etc. are all simple yet good indicators of fitness. Record your results in a journal for later reference.

- Emphasize the pleasurable benefits of exercise. Many people struggle in the beginning, at least until positive changes begin to occur—for example, weight loss or more energy.

- The first four to six weeks of a program can be the most crucial. Reward positive behavior and consistent exercise. Contrary to what many infomercials claim, the benefits don't happen overnight. But I can honestly say they do happen.

- Applaud adherence. More is not better. Keep exercise intensity down and exercise more frequently. If each workout is a grueling ordeal that results in great pain the morning after, how long will you continue to do it? Replace the old adage "no pain, no gain" with "train, don't strain."

Depression is one of the most treatable mental disorders. Because of feelings of fatigue and hopelessness, physical activity can be challenging, but you should make an honest attempt. Exercise can ease the symptoms of depression. A recent Duke University study even found that while the antidepressant drug Prozac eased symptoms more quickly, sixteen weeks down the road, people who exercised three times a week experienced symptom relief similar to those individuals who took Prozac. Even in extreme cases, exercise, combined with therapy and medication, can allow one to enjoy a better quality of life.

— Sean M. Kenney, C.P.T.

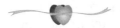

Perspectives on Caregiving

— An Interview with Dana Reeve

Like many of us, **Dana Reeve** became a caregiver overnight. Her husband, actor and director Christopher Reeve, was left paralyzed from the neck down as a result of a riding accident in 1995. Nothing would be the same for the whole family, but the Reeves have learned and grown from this experience.

Gary Barg: How did you explain to your son, Will, about Chris's accident?

Dana Reeve: As a parent, I firmly believe that we need to be as honest as we can with our children, tempering what we say to match the age level of the child. Children are extremely resilient. I think if they feel safe, then you're giving them the best possible tool any parent could give a child: to be able to cope with life's inevitable difficulties.

At first, Will [he was three years old] was afraid of even seeing Chris, but he adapted very quickly. Will repeatedly fell off his hobby horse in the pediatric ward playroom and said, "Oh, my neck, my neck!" I would have to tell him that his neck was fine and that "Daddy's neck is broken and he can't move." We would do this over and over again. It was sort of like play therapy that he was devising on his own.

GB: How have the past three years changed your perspective on life?

DR: I don't take anything for granted. I'm also more cynical and more pragmatic. I don't take a romantic view of life at all anymore; I really take a practical view of life. I don't necessarily see that as a loss, but I do see it as a difference. "Happily ever after" is like "ha-ha-ha."

However, the other side of that is entering into a world where you see the gift behind disability. I mean, it's not as frivolous. There's an intensity to life and relationships that in many ways is extremely fulfilling. I think there's a lot of truth to the adage, "What doesn't kill you makes you stronger."

I'm also finding that you can find joy in the oddest of places and activities. Just in small things. We were looking at the stars the other night, and the idea that

Chris can be out of bed, and the stars were out, and it was so clear with the most beautiful breeze...you just appreciate you're alive, and you're able to look at the stars, and everybody is healthy at the moment. I think that helps us appreciate our family relationship even more.

GB: What has helped you get through these times?

DR: Therapy. I'm a big believer in therapy if you have someone very, very good and qualified. There are some things that I don't think are helpful to share with your spouse. I do think a bad therapist is worse than none at all, but there are wonderful clinical psychologists out there. I consider it to be similar to getting a heart doctor for your heart. A therapist is an emotion doctor for your emotions.

GB: How do you deal with stress?

DR: Stress is an ongoing problem. I find yoga is really helpful, but then I find my life gets so stressed out that I don't have time for yoga. No time for the cure. It's ironic, one of the things I speak on is nurturing the nurturer. I really believe in it. I was telling a friend of mine that I was going to speak on it, and she looked at me and said, "Better start practicing what you preach." I do think you can deal with stress in little ways, you can give yourself little getaways, and it doesn't always have to cost money. It's really a gift you have to give yourself: mini-respites.

GB: What do you do for your "mini-respites"?

DR: Yoga is great when I take the time. But even when I don't, I would just go up into a room where no one will come in and do whatever it takes, whether it's reading, sitting completely quietly, or doing something where I'm not reporting to someone: not answering the phone, not getting something for someone, just locking myself away. Taking a bubble bath, even a mental bubble bath.

GB: **What's been your best source of reliable information as a caregiver?**

DR: Other caregivers. Over the past few years, I've talked to a lot of women whose husbands are injured, sharing tips and ideas and venting to one another. You get advice from your doctors, or you get the official recommended procedure on some things, and then someone else will come in and say, "Oh, you know what's easier?" Or she'd say, "Well, yes, you can spend all this money on this particular kind of bandage, or you can cut up a Maxi pad, and it sticks to the sock." I get all of this useful information about so many different products that are helpful. Everything from machines to suppositories.

GB: **How do you redefine normality in your life?**

DR: I think it becomes easier as you become used to it. The first-year anniversary is very, very tough because every landmark we hit, I remember the year before when it wasn't that way. The second anniversary was easier, because I was looking back on the first year and how tough that was. Then this past year went by, and we've been able to look back and think, "We've come really far. Things are becoming positive and definitely different."

But, there's also some wonderful stuff that comes out of it. I mean meeting people we might never have met and, strangely enough, opportunities that might never have been taken advantage of. Directing is something Chris has always talked about, and then he ended up directing a beautiful film that came directly out of people wanting to reach out and give him opportunities. And he ended up winning awards for it. So, that's something that has come directly out of the tragedy. I'm also grateful for what Chris's injury has done in terms of elevating the consciousness of the country, and the world, about the disabled. He's made a tremendous change in terms of people's awareness.

GB: You must hear all the time about how heroic you've been. How do you feel about that?

DR: I'm actually very uncomfortable with that title because I don't feel like a hero. When Chris and I got married, I took my wedding vows very seriously. When I took those vows and said I would be there in sickness and in health, no matter what, that was the scary day. That was the day when I said, "Okay, here we go. We're going on this journey, and let's hope it's a fun one." Really, it has been.

As far as my situation today, I don't see any other choice. I don't say that in a negative way, it's just not a situation where there is a choice. I'm so grateful that I have the stuff to be able to cope with difficult times. I credit my parents for that. But let's be honest, we have financial resources that many, many people don't have. I was very happy living a kind of an obscure existence. Then suddenly Chris is in the lime-light. The upside of that is that I get support in droves, so I don't see myself as particularly heroic.

I do see many, many caregivers, mostly women, every day, who are the real heroes. People who really have to struggle, who are invisible and not in the limelight. Their husbands are irrevocably depressed and have not been able to get back to work. These women are doing what I'm doing, but have a job that is a thousand times harder. If people say I'm a hero, I'm glad they think, "okay, caregiver equals hero." But, personally, I have it much easier than many people, and I certainly do this out of love and commitment. I also recognize that there's a trap in the perception of caregivers: We do these things out of love and, therefore, we have to do it without any rights. I don't think that's fair.

GB: Chris mentioned in *Still Me* that only 30 percent of people fight their insurance company. Do you have any advice for the other 70 percent?

DR: Yes. My first piece of advice is, "Don't take it personally." When I first started fighting the insurance company, I used to scream and cry, "How can they be doing this to us?" Then I realized they do it to everybody.

My second piece of advice is, when people ask what they can do to help, assign them the task of writing letters to the insurance companies after you get denials. Writing resubmissions becomes an incredibly valuable thing that someone can do for you. It's amazing how much it eases your mind. Whenever someone asks if they can help me, I ask them to do something specific, and it gets done. I think people want to help, even busy people.

GB: Tell me about the Christopher Reeve Foundation.

DR: The mission of the foundation is twofold: to support scientific research toward a cure for paralysis, and to give out what we call Quality of Life grants. These are for people with disabilities in the areas of caregiving, transportation, recreation, personal needs—all different things. We can't give to individuals, but we do give to grassroots organizations. Currently we give $700,000 in grants to organizations, including the National Family Caregivers Association. We're a tiny foundation, and we don't have a big staff. A lot of our fund raising has been just by people sending in money and earmarking it for the foundation.

GB: What positive things do you see in motion for care-givers?

DR: One of the most positive things is that the National Family Caregivers Association was able to get care-givers included in the year 2000 Census. I see that as a very positive step. As caregivers we're working primarily out of a feeling of love and obligation toward the person for whom we care. But that's also when we become invisible. We don't see it as a job, it's just part of our life. But it is a job and there should be tax breaks, as well as other kinds of assistance. Also, the amount of money family caregivers are saving the health care system is tremendous. It's phenomenal, and this is something I don't think people realize. We have to speak out and be counted in a census.

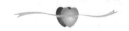

Chapter 8

Care of the Caregiver

Always There

Your loving parents were always there for you
Little league, cheerleading, school and even after
Caring, sharing and guiding you through
Windstorms, rainstorms, whatever disaster.

Protecting, nurturing, surrounding you in love,
Giving you a feeling you can never describe
A feeling you can make it, always rise above
A high much greater than any drug can devise.

Now you're a parent sharing life anew
With your children bonding as you once did,
So the cycle of life continues with you
Waking memories of childhood once hid.

Minds wander to days when the cycle reversed
Always there for your parents, returning the love,
Spontaneous actions, nothing rehearsed,
A giving returned and now they're above.

You hope your children can someday feel
The warmth and loving that you did share,
Sensations that now almost seem unreal
All stemming from that need to always be there.

— Gary Slavin

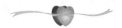

Prisoners of Compassion

Henry Nouwen suggested that those involved in the helping professions, whether clergy, nurses, or what have you,
are wounded healers. That title seems particularly appropriate for those who are caregivers because, so frequently,
such persons are prisoners of compassion.

The very word *compassion* comes from the Latin and
means "with suffering" or "suffering with." Caregivers, by
the very nature of the tasks they face daily, truly suffer with
those for whom they care. The bonds may be those of volun-
tary love, for love is always costly: it demands expression. On
the other hand, they may be the bonds of obligatory responsibility. The caregiver is stuck with these duties because no one
else is prepared or willing to help. In either case, one can become a prisoner of compassion. The vital difference is one
of perspective.

Caregivers should look at how they view themselves. Their
self-image is crucial when it comes to the power to cope.
Your outlook can make you bitter or better. My experience
in working with caregivers over several decades drives this
fact home. Caregivers tend to look on their lives as either a
gift or an *entitlement*. If they look on their life as an entitlement, something due them just because they were born,

then every difficult situation, accident, disease, physical or emotional setback is seen as an unwelcome and undeserved intrusion on their much-deserved happiness. Such people typically become critical, cynical, and bitter. They tend to blame God, the physicians, even the person for whom they care, for their own bitter fate. They view life as fundamentally unfair.

On the other hand, there are those who look on life as a gift, a boon, something so splendid and undeserved that every breath is a blessing and every hour an honor. Such people may begin each day as a caregiver friend who prays at each day's beginning: "Good morning, dear God. This is your day, I am your child, have your own way." People with that kind of outlook tend to reach out naturally to others less fortunate, thankful that they can do so. As early Christians explained their remarkable capacity to show love: "We love, because He first loved us."

All of us who would help others do so as wounded healers. Our task is not easy, but it is needful. We are at our best when we begin each day with gratitude, offering thanks for yet another day in which to receive and offer love. It isn't always easy; it is always necessary if we—and those we care for—are to become better and not bitter.

— Dr. Gerald Trigg

Caregiver Burnout

Being able to cope with the stress of being a caregiver is part of the art of caregiving. To remain healthy so that we can continue to be caregivers, we must be able to recognize our own limitations and learn to care for ourselves and others.

It is important for all of us to try to recognize the signs of burnout. To do this we must be honest and willing to hear feedback from those around us. This is especially important for those caring for family or friends. Too often caregivers who are not closely associated with the health care profession are overlooked and get lost in the commotion of medical emergencies and procedures. Otherwise close friends begin to grow distant, and eventually the caregiver is alone without a support structure. We must allow those who do care for us, who are interested enough to say something, to tell us about our behavior—for example, a noticeable decrease in energy or mood changes.

Burnout isn't like a cold. You don't always notice it when you are in its clutches. Very much like post-traumatic stress disorder, the symptoms of burnout can begin surfacing months after a traumatic episode. The following are symptoms we might notice in ourselves, or others might say they see in us:

- feelings of depression,
- a sense of ongoing and constant fatigue,
- decreasing interest in work,
- decrease in work production,
- withdrawal from social contacts,
- increasing use of stimulants and alcohol,
- increasing fear of death,
- change in eating patterns, or
- feelings of helplessness.

Strategies to ward off or cope with burnout are important. To counteract burnout, the following specific strategies are recommended:

- Participate in a support network.
- Consult with professionals to explore burnout issues.
- Attend a support group to receive feedback and coping strategies.
- Vary the focus of caregiving responsibilities if possible (rotate responsibilities with family members).
- Exercise daily and maintain a healthy diet.
- Establish quiet time for meditation.
- Get a weekly massage.
- Stay involved in hobbies.

By acknowledging the reality that being a caregiver is filled with stress and anxiety, and understanding the potential for burnout, caregivers can be forewarned and can guard against this debilitating condition. As much as it is said, it still cannot be said too often: The best way to be an effective caregiver is to take care of yourself.

— Dr. M. Ross Seligson

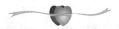

Respite: Enjoy a Guilt-Free Time-Out

Why is it that the words *respite* and *guilt* seem to go hand in hand? Why do we as caregivers feel we are somehow failing our loved one by admitting that we need help, need time to recharge our batteries, or just need time to play a bit? Perhaps because so many of us still hold on to the myth that says the caregiver has to be all things to all people.

The truth is, no matter how we try, we are not caregivers *extraordinaire*. We are human, with all the same needs and feelings as everyone else. And, just like everyone else, we need to take time to smell the roses.

For many caregivers, the thought of going away for even a brief time is fraught with fears of disaster and chaos because we are not there to oversee everything. After all, we all know that no one can replace what we do as caregivers for our family member or loved one.

And this belief is not so far from the truth. In fact, I still believe firmly that no one can replace the caregiver. The love and support we provide to our charge cannot be duplicated by anyone. Still, sometimes, it is okay to let someone else do the best he or she can for our family member, so that we can take time to regroup and, in doing so, be able to continue to be the wonderful caregivers we have been. It is a simple concept when you think about it. In using the principles of respite we ultimately will be providing the very best care that is humanly possible to our loved one.

As caregivers it is important that we recognize that it is okay to take a break from our caregiving duties. It is okay to feel tired and want a break from caregiving. Not only is it okay, it is your right. You are allowed to stay healthy physically and emotionally. Actually, by not doing so you are helping to create a potential problem down the road. No one can keep going day after day without a break; sooner or later it is going to catch up with you, and not only will you suffer, but your loved one will as well. It is equally important to know that not taking that break can and often does result in medical complications to the caregiver. If a medical emergency develops for caregivers, who helps to care for their loved one?

Ask caregivers who have been at it for any length of time, and you will learn that their own health has suffered when they failed to take proper care of themselves. Respite care is one way the caregiver can get this needed break and, one hopes, do it without guilt. By taking care of yourself and recharging your own batteries, you are ultimately taking care of your loved one. There is no need to allow guilt into the picture. All that will do is prevent you from reaping the full rewards of a true respite.

Respite care can be anything from a few hours a week to longer periods of up to two weeks or longer to provide care to a loved one while the caregiver takes a break. Respite care provides caregivers the opportunity to:

- take a vacation,

- have a weekend getaway,

- attend to home or work responsibilities that have been building up, or

- recharge their energy to be better prepared to provide the attention and patience required daily.

Think about these principles to ensure your guilt-free respite:

- I am entitled to take care of myself.

- I am worthy of a break.

- I am showing my commitment to my caregiver role when I take steps like respite care to ensure that continued quality care is delivered to my loved one.

- It is okay to relax and enjoy other aspects of my life.

- It is okay to take a break and recharge my energies.
- It is okay to maintain as much normalcy in my life as possible.
- It is okay to continue to dream.

If roles were reversed, there is no question I would want my loved one to have a respite. It is right and responsible of me to have a respite as well.

Respite Solutions

Some short-term respite solutions include enlisting another family member, neighbor, or friend to stay with your loved one for a few hours several times a week. This offers an opportunity for you, the caregiver, to have a mini-respite to shop, go to a movie, get your hair done, even have a pampering facial. For many who are not comfortable leaving their family member for longer than a few hours, this is an excellent way to recharge the batteries and, at the same time, do something special for yourself.

Often it is just doing a little something extra like this that can make all the difference to caregivers who are feeling the strain of all they have to do each day.

Another option, one that I highly recommend to all caregivers, is the scheduled respite in which your loved one is entrusted into the care of a respite service center, or perhaps another family member can take on the role while you have a much needed rest. Respite centers offer temporary residents a variety of services that meet all of their needs. These centers offer myriad services, from around-the-clock medical care to recreational activities, and vacationing family members can relax knowing that their loved one is well taken care of during their absence.

You can locate respite centers or respite services in your area by contacting your local agency on aging. That organization can direct you to any services available and provide information on what Medicare and Medicaid will cover. Another resource might be your religious community. Your local social service agency, the local Alzheimer's association, Easter Seals, or mental health agency offices are all resources that can help you to find the right respite care.

So go ahead and plan for the respite caregivers so richly deserve and need. You will be glad you did, and if you have not had a respite before, you are going to wonder what took you so long.

— Catherine Murphy, R.N.

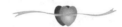

20 Ways for Caregivers to Take Care of Themselves

1. Laugh about something every day.

2. Take care of yourself physically.

3. Eat a well-balanced diet.

4. Talk with someone every day.

5. Let family and friends help. Give them printed material explaining what you are dealing with so they can better understand your loved one. Give them a chance.

6. Give yourself permission to have a good cry. Tears aren't a weakness; they reduce tension.

7. Exercise—a brisk walk counts.

8. Get adequate rest.

9. Try a bowl of Cheerios and milk before bed to promote sleep.

10. Avoid tension-filled and/or noisy movies at night. The late news itself can add to your stress, so skip it.

11. Reduce your daily caffeine intake.

12. Get professional help if your support system isn't adequate or if you feel overwhelmed.

13. Take a break every day, even if it's only ten minutes alone in the backyard.

14. Explore community resources and connect with them.

15. Listen to music.

16. Learn relaxation techniques.

17. Attend one or more support groups and education workshops regularly.

18. Give yourself a treat at least once a month: an ice cream cone, a new shirt or dress, a night out with friends, a flowering plant.

19. Read your Caregiver's Bill of Rights (see chapter 1).

20. Know your limitations.

— *Today's Caregiver Magazine*

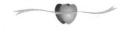

Take Regular Breaks

You must remember to take regular breaks from your caregiving responsibilities. You can't be good to someone else if you're not good to yourself. Use your relatives. They can help in several ways—financially, socially, and as respite. If relatives are unavailable, try community services like a volunteer group at your local church.

Follow these guidelines for caregiving breaks:

- Every day, take a half-hour to do something you like that is relaxing: practice yoga, meditate, do needlepoint, read.
- Every week, spend a couple of hours away from the house at a place you like: a museum, theater, mall, coffeehouse, library.
- Every month, spend an evening out with friends, go to a play or concert, a movie, or a restaurant.
- Every year, go on a well-planned (and well-deserved) vacation.

These guidelines will help to avoid caregiver burnout.

— Michael Plontz

Top Ten Ways to Care for Yourself

1. **Find all related information on caregiving.** Community resources such as libraries, hospitals, and local health care agencies can supply you with appropriate books, brochures and magazines as well as contact information for local support organizations.

2. **Be practical with the goals you set for your loved one and yourself.** Learn to set priorities and stress the importance of family involvement to help you meet your needs and carry out the daily activities of caregiving. When people ask whether they can help, give them specific tasks with which you need help.

3. **Understand that caregiving is often a stressful activity.** Certain aspects of caregiving are more stressful than others, but planning proper responses ahead of time can reduce your stress and improve your overall emotional state. Try not to be critical of yourself in moments of stress or irritation.

4. **Stay in touch with your friends and as much as possible, do not give up being involved in activities that you enjoy.** To offer your loved one the best care possible, you must also focus on your own happiness and well being.

5. **Take advantage of respite services available for you and your loved one.** Home care aides are available to help you provide care for your loved one, if needed. For assistance during the days while you are at work, investigate options available at senior daycare facilities,

local churches, and community centers that offer supervision and daily activities.

6. **Keep a caregiver journal.** Writing things down not only helps you better track your loved one's medical care but also allows you an opportunity to review your daily goals and successes.

7. **Daily relaxation methods such as laughter and exercise can provide a welcome relief.** Choose an appropriate exercise regimen to follow, such as walking or attending classes at a local gym, to help alleviate frustrations and emotional discomfort. Remembering to include laughter in your life is not always easy, but watching a comedy on television with your loved one or visiting with friends may present you with some much needed moments of joy.

8. **Focus on improving communication with your loved one, family, and friends.** If possible, allow your loved one to have a role in his or her own care, ask others for advice, and be willing to listen to their opinions. Do not be afraid to ask people for any support that they may be able to offer.

9. **Join a caregiver support group.** This forum allows caregivers to learn better coping strategies. Going to a support groups does not mean you are an inadequate caregiver; rather, it can improve your relationship with your loved one and provide an outlet for you to freely speak your mind with people who understand what you are going through.

10. **Concentrate on your own mental and physical health.** Eating properly, getting enough rest, and allowing for your "personal time" can go a long way toward balancing

the act of caregiving with your overall health. If you lost your health and stamina, who else would have the compassion and courage to step in and provide care for both you and your loved one?

— *Today's Caregiver Magazine*

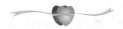

Tips and Techniques for Dealing with Stress

Change is an expected part of our daily lives today. Dealing with it so that you control it rather than it controlling you is an important and positive force. Try a few of these tips.

- Accept what you cannot change. Take a tip from Alcoholics Anonymous. Change what you can, if it bothers you. But, if you cannot change it, learn to live with it.

- Face up to your problems. Sort them out, and see which ones are real and which are simply imagined. Deal with them as they are, not as what you think they are.

- Deal with one problem at a time. Sort out your priorities, and deal with them in the order of their importance to you.

- Be flexible. Give in once in a while. If you do, others will too.

- Don't hold all of your worries inside yourself—talk them out. Frequently we swallow our unhappiness (along with candy, cake, ice cream, etc.) because we can't let the problems out. Talk to someone. A burden shared is much less of a burden.

- Work off stress. Physical outlets for stress help your body fight off many of the negative results of stress.

- Get enough rest/relaxation/sleep. Give your body a chance to recover from day to day. Lack of sleep will only make matters worse for you.

- Avoid self-medication. A spoonful of sugar may make the medicine go down, but it does your body no good. Sugar, alcohol, nicotine, and ice cream may all feel good going down, but they make matters worse—from the inside. They add to your body's physical stresses, thus making dealing with external stresses much harder.

- Take time to smell the roses. Have some fun. Relax.

- Think about and do something for others. A little altruism never hurt; it even makes people feel better about themselves.

- Be the captain of your ship. If you are not happy with your life, think about what's wrong or missing, and then plan the necessary actions to change it to coincide with your needs and what you want for your life.

- Work on your relationships with those who share your life. Don't hold back your feelings. Share them with your family, friends, and coworkers. It can help to decrease tensions.

— Dr. Rita Nachen Gugel

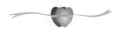

Write Your Way to Better Health

Good news! A scientifically proven method for relieving stress is, literally, within your grasp: grab a pen and write. But not just any type of writing will do. It's not enough to list your complaints. You need to reflect on your situation and explore your thoughts and feelings in depth in a process called *expressive writing.*

In the 1980s, Dr. James W. Pennebaker's research discovered that writing deep thoughts and feelings about traumatic events calmed people down, improved their moods and outlook, and increased lymphocytes, white cells that boost the immune system. When he analyzed the contents of their writing, Dr. Pennebaker found that as people wrote more and more about stressful events, they came to a deeper understanding of their upsets. In fact, he found that not writing or talking about upsetting events could be unhealthy.

"But I'm Not a Writer!"

Even if the only writing you do is the checks to pay bills, you can do expressive writing. You don't have to share your words with anyone; you write for your eyes only. Spelling, grammar, and punctuation don't matter. What matters is that you explore your thoughts and feelings in words, and that you, as Dr. Pennebaker says, "translate your emotional experiences into language."

Expressive writing is a mental process that helps you integrate information and experiences. It is a flexible activity that you can do anywhere and anytime. Writing in this way allows you to gain perspective on your situation and understand events in your life.

While there is no right or wrong way to begin a writing exploration, it can be frustrating to sit down with a blank piece of paper or computer screen and not know where to begin. To avoid that frustration, create a list of writing topics that you want to address and add to the list whenever you think of a new one. As you write your narratives, more topics will come to you. While each person's caregiving experience is unique, many writing topics are common to all. Here are a few:

- How do you feel about the person in your care?
- What concerns have you had about money or insurance?
- What good things have you experienced from being a caregiver?
- What disagreements have you had with the person in your care over issues of control?
- Are you able to talk openly and honestly with the person in your care about his or her condition and prognosis?
- Who else in your family has had this condition, and how does repetition of this similar condition affect you?

When you embark on an expressive writing session, you might consider treating it as a sacred time by lighting a candle, which in many cultures is a symbol of the search for meaning. To tune out distractions and noise, close your eyes and take a deep breath. Breathe deeply again. Tell yourself you have nothing more important to do at this moment. Still with your eyes closed, think of the topic you'll be writing about. Then open your eyes and write. Don't censor yourself; write whatever comes to mind.

Your writing medium is a personal choice. Many people prefer pen and paper for this type of writing because they can almost feel their thoughts turn into words as the connection is made from hand to pen to paper. There is the temptation on a computer to rewrite at length, to chisel and hone your writing into a perfect piece of prose. You eventually may decide to give your work to someone else to read, or even publish it, but you are the audience for this writing, at least in its first draft stage.

Writing to heal may bring up feelings you may not feel prepared to handle alone. A certain amount of upset is expected because this type of writing requires deep emotional honesty. However, if you find that what you write is too emotionally upsetting, see a mental health counselor to help you deal with your feelings.

Expressive writing can free your mind of recurring thoughts and feelings that keep you from appreciating other facets of your life. So, write! Write to release stress and boost your immune system.

— Margie Davis

Backing away from Hell

— An Interview with Mariette Hartley

Currently, Emmy award–winning actress **Mariette Hartley** is hosting her fifth season of the acclaimed *Healthy Solutions* television series. You can visit the Web site at www.healthysolutions.tv.

As national spokesperson for the American Foundation for Suicide Prevention, Mariette was honored with its humanitarian award for her outstanding work in the field of suicide prevention and research. She is also involved with the Center to Prevent Handgun Violence, SOJOURN, and M.A.D.D.

Gary Barg: When did you first see yourself as a caregiver?

Mariette Hartley: I've been a caregiver since I was a child. I was always the one that friends would talk to. I was very much my parents' parent on some level. I see a lot of caregivers who are very unhappy and nurture themselves in self-destructive ways, and I think a lot of that is because they didn't have a childhood on some level. Often we're also forced into caregiving at too early an age. I've had time to back up and give myself that time, or if I find myself harassed during a particular day, I now know that it's time for me to get very quiet and to nurture myself.

GB: Do you think that one of the things that caregivers never do is take care of themselves?

MH: That's right. Absolutely, and it's a deceptively destructive way to live because it keeps the focus off ourselves and then we don't take the tests that we need to take. Yes, you're absolutely right. They don't take care of themselves. And there's a balance. There's definitely a balance. I mean there were days with my mother when I was exhausted. There will be days when caregivers will be exhausted. But we need to balance that then with something that will give care to us in order to be able to go back in there and get back into the battle.

GB: Your mother died of emphysema. Can you tell me about taking care of her?

MH: She lived in my house until three months before she died and it was very, very hard. I paid for a full-time nurse to be there, and I wanted her to die in that house if she needed to, but it was terribly disruptive. So I found a wonderful apartment about two blocks away from me and I was then able to give her better care. I was able to come in every day. Be with her every day, and it was such a brilliant time for the two of us because my mother allowed herself to be taken care of for the first time in her life. Really taken care of. It was the first time that my mother and I held one another without one of us letting go. And that was because of the way she had been raised, and I wrote about this because I felt it was important that my mother always used to pull away. I would come to her for a hug and she would pull away, and she told me that she did that because she didn't want me to become too dependent.

GB: **Your situation is similar to what many of our readers are going through.**

MH: Well, they must go through it. And they must go through it as present as they can be because it is a gift. My mother died in my brother's and my arms. We brought the entire family around, and she ultimately turned off her own air because she was in agony and she was going through dementia. So, we watched it and supported her. We had to. What else can you do at that point? She knew she had about three days to live and so did my husband and it was amazing. It was a celebration of a passing and my mother taught me more almost in her death than she did in her life. Although as I sort through our lives together I see that she gave me extraordinary gifts, it was so mixed with so much other stuff, it was really difficult to sort out. Her death was clear, pure, dignified. I was able to give to her completely. I was sober and I have been sober for a long time now, so there was nothing that anesthetized any of that. I was so present for it. I remember it vividly and it was an extraordinary experience, and she was funny—I'll never forget it. She woke up after she had turned off her air. She woke up at 4:00 in the morning. She said, "What time is it?" I said, "It's 4:00, mom." She said, "I'm not dead yet?" I said, "No, honey, you're not dead yet."

GB: What would you tell a caregiver who is facing the imminent death of his or her loved one?

MH: People need to know that first of all they're not alone in it. I was so grateful that I had enough money to be able to support her through it and to have her live in a style to which she was accustomed. It was a beautiful little apartment. It was an extraordinary, detailed, loving experience for all of us and I would wish that on anybody. If the family is around, it becomes a totally inclusive experience. Having experienced that myself, there is nothing like it. It's like a birth. It's like a home birth. It's exactly the same, you know. We catch the baby and we pass the baby on.

GB: How did you deal with the grief when your mother died?

MH: We need to share our grief with people. I would certainly recommend support groups. I deeply believe in support groups of all kinds. I mean if somebody for example is a drinker and is drinking through the death of a parent and finds themselves drinking more and more and more, you know, get to a twelve-step program. It's the answer as far as I'm concerned. If it's a parent who has lost a child, Compassionate Friends has a wonderful program. They have candlelight services. They really know how to serve loss and loss is something that we have to learn, unfortunately. I mean a lot of us think that the grieving process is fast. That we should be able to get through it just like that. There are things you can do to get through it. You can read books to elderly people who are still alive and desperately need that. You can play the piano for Jewish Homes, and give that pain meaning. I mean, that's what my life is all about today. And as frightening as that was for me, because I do believe that many of us get to heaven by backing away from hell, if I were to have a message of my life, it's that one's deepest pain integrated becomes one's greatest power. And we have to find that power. We have to, and it's in finding the power that the integration begins. And it takes time but I have been through it, and people know that I mean what I say because I've walked through the fire. I've been helped through the fire. People have put their hand to me over the River Styx and have pulled me over, so that's what I get to do now. I reach and help other people who are not in such good shape and help them. I know the journey. I would recommend helping others to anybody who knows that journey.

GB: What can you tell caregivers about stress?

MH: Look, I have no research and I don't know how much research there is out there and I'm hoping that our organization will be able to do this. What is the research out there on what stress does biochemically to us? What does it do to the serotonin level in the brain? My hunch is that it has an enormous effect. I'm certainly one of the people that will tell you that it does. We need to take care of ourselves. What I always say—and I mean it with every part of my being—

when you are on a plane what does the stewardess say to you? What does the attendant say to you when the oxygen comes down?

GB: **Put it on your own face first.**

MH: That's right—then put it on your child's face. Well, your parent is your child. Whatever you can do that's humanly possible to help her, you must do. But you also must take care of yourself. If it means spending a day in a spa, don't say, "My God, I couldn't do that!" Not only can you do that, you must! Even if it's having a friend give you a massage, if you can't afford it. Have someone rub your feet. Buy some candles. Take a nice warm bath. Meditate. Eat well. You have to take care of yourself because once the person's gone, there's you. You have your life then. My God, if you don't have a life, what do you go back to? It's like when my mother used to say, we'd go to parties and I'd say, "Mom, I'm so nervous about it," and she'd say, "Just be yourself, honey." To myself I'd say, "What is me, I don't know who I am." I've come to know who I am now. And I think that's the other thing that happens to us. We only feel that way because we aren't taking care of ourselves. We're allowing people to suck us dry, and we can't do it. If it means going to church, find a church that you love. Find a spiritual base that you love. That's why the twelve-step programs are so amazing. Al Anon is an amazing program based on the twelve-step programs. I am powerless over people, places, and things. Hello! Caregivers think that they can come in like the Michelin Man, with their God suit in place and save the world. You can't.

GB: **What should caregivers do to balance caregiving and keep up with their own lives?**

MH: In my case I had another life. My life was filled with work or with my husband, with my children, with adopted children, with neighborhood children, with kids that call me mom all over the country, so I definitely had a life when it was time for my mother to go. If it's your only life—and I think that does happen with certain people—then you really need to find a life, if we're to be happy, healthy people. If we're to have our own lives.

Chapter 9

Caregivers and the Holidays

A Caregiver's Christmas

'Twas the night before Christmas, when all through the
   house
a caregiver was scurrying, caring for her dear spouse;
His stockings were placed upon his feet with great care
in hopes he felt well enough to step out for some fresh
   air.
Their children were scattered, all snug in their beds
around this great country, not a care in their heads.
And the caregiver who worked nightshift, 'cause the
   funds they did tap
had just settled down for a five-minute nap,
When in the next room, there arose such a clatter,
she sprang from her bed to see what did splatter.
Away past the bedsheets she had thrown in the trash,
tore open a new set and hoped these would last.
The weight on her breast was of one who did know
that by the luster of daybreak, her sorrow would grow.

When, what in any other year would be a thing quite so
    dear
that time when her family would visit from far and
    from near.
With no one to hold her, since her loved one took sick,
she felt that the holidays were just a mean trick.
More rapid than eagles her friends they did flee
When they could no longer travel or even take tea.
No Cohens! No Schwartzes! No Millers! No Dicksons!
No Olivets! No Lutids, no Donners or Micksons.
For a while they gave support, for a while did they call,
"Now dash away! Dash away! Dash away to the mall!"
As new restaurants that before were easy to try,
when her loved one was too sick, away did they fly.
So now with the holidays, the family will do
with the sleigh full of presents and bad advice, too.
And then, in a twinkling, I heard in the drive
Aunt Nancy and Chloe and all my in-laws arrive.
As I had in my hand, a bedpan disposal bound
I turned very quickly and tripped over the hound.
My man was a mess from his head to his toes,
and his clothes were soiled and not easy on the nose.
A bundle of nerves, I shout out very loud,
words, which to this day, do not make me feel proud.
He lies there so quiet, not saying a thing
when suddenly his laughter filled our home like a fresh
    breath of spring.
He doubled over with glee making such a roil
that he slapped a bad knee through the all-too-grim soil.
As his eyes twinkled through all the great mess, this old
    dear,
For a moment, I forgot the pain of this past year.
On a normal night, the pain of his stump would make
    him tighten his teeth,

but tonight, for a moment, his laughter caused such
  uncommon relief.
That the joy of it encircled his head like a wreath;
as he lay on the bed, he shook his round belly,
for all the world, not unlike a big bowl of jelly.
He was lying there laughing, like a jolly old elf,
and I laughed when I saw him, in spite of myself.
When, all of a sudden, the door burst open wide as
  can be,
and what did I see, but the Cohens, the Schwartzes,
  and Aunt Nancy all looking at me.
With nary a word they made up the bed
Then they all straightened up and got us both fed.
They all had not known the support that I needed,
but once they saw they could help, they learned and
  succeeded
In sharing the heart, the soul, and the care
That I always was sure were really right there.
I hadn't spoken a word of the great strain and the
  work
That I thought they had all turned into one major jerk.
After knowing what help each could give if I asked,
I never alone had to shoulder the entire task.
We had time to play and to sing and to wet a whistle
until away they all flew like the down of a thistle.
But I heard my loved ones, as they drove out of sight:
"Happy Christmas to all, and to all a good-night!
And, we're coming back next Friday eve to take you
  for a bite."

— Gary Barg

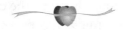

Nourishing Holidays

Ah, 'tis the season...But for many of us, it is another day of the same old thing, or, maybe worse, it is a time when even more expectations and responsibilities are placed on us than we usually face. Maybe they come from inside, or maybe they are the expectations of others. Nonetheless, the holiday season can be more burdensome than joyful for many of us.

One hopes you can make some time for yourself for inner reflection—some time to consider things or people for whom you are grateful and some things that you would like to do a little differently in your future.

So, I invite you to consider your relationship with food! Some of you may scratch your head, "Relationship with food? I have relationships with people or pets, not food!" This may be true for the many of us who truly view food as a means of sustenance. But you may know folks who truly don't care what they eat and may even forget to eat, unless someone reminds them or prepares food for them.

There are others of us, however, for whom foods, especially certain foods, seem to have a voice in our heads. It may sound like, "I'm here waiting for you to eat me—please don't leave me in this half-empty bag [or container] in the dark all night" or "Oh, it's the holidays, and we both know I'm not good for you. Still, just this once, a little bit won't hurt."

As a nutritionist, I often speak to people about the nutrients in the food they eat. I am learning more and more that there is a lot more to food than just the chemicals that make up the protein, fat, vitamins, and minerals. In *Nourishing Wisdom,* author Marc David shows how the psychological and spiritual aspects of our lives affect how and if we are truly nurtured. In his book, David suggests that we need to experience food as a neutral thing—no "good" or "bad" food—and listen to our bodies instead to know what to eat.

The foods we humans eat are greatly influenced by our culture and psychology, rather than by our instinct. Our bodies want and need different foods at different times. We prefer salads and light foods in the summer, and soups and heavier foods during the colder, darker winter months. There may be times when we are happy or sad that we want a certain food because it is familiar to us or is associated with similar circumstances in our past.

At holiday times, we look forward to special foods. Why? For many of us, they remind us of happy times, special times, and, perhaps, times when someone else was responsible for the cooking. These special foods have the capacity to nourish us in more ways than just giving us calories and vitamins and minerals because each of us longs to belong, to know we are important to someone or that we have made a difference in someone's life. If, somehow, we are not sure of these things, we may turn to eating certain foods to feel comforted, or to preparing foods for others to be sure we are needed and appreciated.

As we grow older, many of us are faced with chronic diseases such as high blood pressure, heart disease, or diabetes. We may find it harder to maintain our youthful figures; but still, each year the holidays come around, luring us with their many treats that often are not very healthy for us in the long run.

Instead of feeling compelled to eat one more cookie or sliver of pie, and then feel guilty about it, consider this instead. Take a few seconds to ask yourself, "Am I really hungry for this? How will I feel later, if I eat this now?" Or "Do I need it right this minute? Could I wait 'til later when I'm not so full?" It will take just a few seconds and it may save you from feeling bad for a lot longer later. And, as with anything new you try, you will forget sometimes. Do not worry about that! Celebrate the times you remember. Celebrate the times you remember to take care of yourself!

As you are shopping at the bakery or getting out your family's favorite recipes full of butter and sugar, ask yourself, "How can I make this recipe a little healthier—and still taste good? What's important here?" Is it that we have the same foods that taste the same, or is it that we celebrate life and its many pleasures and treasures and challenges this past year has brought? If that's what the holidays are about, then it may not matter what foods are on the table, healthy or not. But it may matter, in the long run, if you feel good about yourself, because you know that taking care of your health and the health of your loved ones is a year-round commitment.

— Rita Miller-Huey, M.Ed., R.D., L.D.

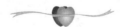

FUN-damental Holiday Stress Busters

Although anyone in any profession can experience increased stress during the holidays, health care professionals are especially vulnerable. They tend to be obsessed with a need to contribute to life through their career dedication.

They have to deal not only with a variety of patients and their families, but also with stressed-out coworkers. Many of them are overburdened and often underappreciated professionals who give 100 percent to their careers. Yet they inevitably lose their creative edge, grow cynical more quickly, burn out faster, and spend just as many holiday working hours pouting as producing.

The following strategies may help to alleviate some of the tightening up that care professionals experience during the holiday season. If you are anything like me, you will probably try all of these approaches at once to have them perfected by the holidays. I advise against such obsession. Such a fanatical approach to lightening up more often leads to tightening up.

Play

Think of the world as a wonderful playground, a giant park full of characters, fantasies, dreams, and love. Learn to play on that playground, to play so hard you lose all sense of time. Many care professionals do not really know what it means to play. They willingly agree, saying, "I play hard and work hard!" However, they do not understand that play is not supposed to be hard; that is why it's called play.

Playing means having fun, at work and at home. We all have to define what play means to us. But, if you have to work at it, you need to evaluate how you see play. Play means spending time inside your body, breathing oxygen, and laughing out loud. Adults who know how to play enjoy belly laughs. They know adult play can be as exciting as playing hide-and-seek when you were a kid. Trust me, there is nothing like a good belly laugh to get the endorphins working.

Do Nothing/Meditate

Sure, it sounds scary, especially during the holiday season. Many of you have tried to meditate or do nothing, but you tried too hard. The little voices in your head bombarded you with stress daily and focused your attention on holiday demands.

It is not easy to learn to do nothing or to meditate, and it often feels so selfish. But, persistence pays off. Start with sixty seconds a day to be truly alone, one full minute to communicate deeply with yourself. After a while this "centering" time can be expanded to three or four minutes to connect with your spirit. We all have a safe place inside ourselves, where our spirit is at rest. Learning to just sit with our feelings can have a profound and comforting effect on our lives.

During the Holidays, Quit Being a Workaholic

There is nothing wrong with dedication to your career or working through the holidays. What does bother me is losing your perspective by placing too much emphasis on work. It is too easy to find yourself out of balance that way. Don't subscribe to myths that claim fun and silliness preclude seriousness, and that somehow humor is unprofessional. There is a great deal of wisdom in the expression *dead serious.* It is well documented that humor is healthy. So take a little time to be silly; you may enjoy it.

Stretch Out to Others

Stretching out to others goes beyond just reaching out. It means delegating and cooperating. It means asking loved ones to reach out, to include you, to pray for you. It means asking colleagues and bosses for conversation, laughter, and direction.

Stretch yourself to make more room for love. Practice stretching yourself by listening, negotiating, and sharing yourself. It will make you flexible and banish your stress. Watch yourself stretch to new heights! In the ever-changing field of health care, failure to practice stress reduction in the workplace undermines productivity, creativity, and adaptability. It literally leads to career suicide (often referred to as burnout.)

— Sherri Issa, M.S.W., L.C.S.W., D.A.B.C.M.

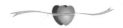

Coping with Holidays as a Caregiver

We all know that holidays can be a very stressful time just in ordinary family life. There is much confusion with the hustle and bustle of preparing for extra company, fixing special meals, and playing the host while trying to enjoy the whole experience as well. For the caregiver, this time can add a whole new set of strains to an already stressful situation.

One of the most important points to remember in our role as caregiver is to try to maintain a sense of familiarity for the one we are caring for. Confusion and change often bring out the worst in us. Imagine, then, what it can do to someone with memory problems, physical impairment, or other handicap. With this in mind, here are some tips that may help make the holidays a little more enjoyable for all involved.

Try to include your loved one in some holiday preparations. Focus on your loved one's remaining strengths, and let that person use his or her own capabilities to help with small tasks. It makes your loved one feel useful, while at the same time helping to occupy him or her while you get on with other preparations. I remember so well having my mom peel the potatoes for me. She enjoyed doing it so much that she peeled ten pounds before I stopped her. She was happy, so I let her go!

With the holidays comes decorating. Try to minimize the amount of clutter this may add.

Whatever holiday you are celebrating, gift giving is an inevitable part of most of the festivities. You might want to consider putting out only a few gifts. There is no need to spread them out so that they fill half the living room. This only creates a hazard for the one you are caring for—by tripping them up or confusing them.

One year my mom felt the need to rearrange all the gifts. We are still missing a few, but we learned from the experience to be selective in how we placed them.

With all of the extra decorating comes the use of additional electrical cords. Be sure to secure all extra cords so they are not a hazard. Try to run them along the outside walls where they are not so visible.

Another good idea is to try to maintain consistent furniture placement. For someone who may be a little confused at times, moving the furniture around may lead to more confusion and agitation.

Also remember to consider the live plants you use in your decorating schemes; be sure to avoid placing poisonous plants on display. Using beautiful artificial flowers is a safer way to make a room colorful.

Try to schedule major activities early in the day. We know that as the day wears on, we all become tired under normal conditions. For someone who is struggling to find his or her place in an already confusing world, stress and agitation increase as the day goes on. Saving time for sitting and visiting quietly toward the end of the day benefits all concerned. Talking about past holiday customs and recipes may be enjoyable for your loved one, especially if he or she has long-term memory recall.

Try to limit the number of guests so there isn't too much hubbub. Keep in mind that the more noise, the more confusion there will be. If your holiday activities are planned well in advance, each guest should be made aware of the emotional state of the one you are caring for. You could even send your guests material to read giving them an overview of the disease if they are unaware of what it entails. This would also be an excellent opportunity to prepare friends and family for the changes they might see in your loved one, especially if they have not been to visit in some time.

Most important, always try to make your loved one feel secure and protected. As much as possible keep him or her on his or her regular routine. We all know that even a slight change in routine can increase confusion and stress. Your holiday plans will flow a lot more smoothly if everyone is aware of your loved one's needs and limitations.

With guests in and out of the house, be sure that someone is aware at all times of where your loved one is. If he or she tends to wander, there is a chance that this may happen while everyone thinks that someone else is watching Aunt Mary! It may be a good idea to assign different people to take turns keeping your loved one in sight. And if your loved one becomes agitated, try to remove him or her to a quiet area of the house, either with you or with someone your loved one trusts. Your loved one could be trying to tell you that he or she needs a break from the activities.

Finally, be sure to fit some time in for yourself this holiday season. If you have extra people there, use them to your advantage. Take a few minutes sometime during the day to pamper yourself! Remember, this is your holiday, too, and do not be afraid to let family know that a little quiet time for yourself would be a gift beyond measure. Place your sister or brother in charge of Mom or Dad or your husband and go run yourself a hot bubble bath or take a thirty-minute much-needed nap. Something this simple will refresh you and help you to enjoy the holidays that much more.

— Brenda Race

Healthy Holiday Recipe

Each of us has our own expectations for the holidays. As a youth, I thought it was supposed to be like in the movies. My family had some strange holiday habits, though, like the year my parents painted the kitchen on Christmas Eve. I was always disappointed.

As a young adult I lived in Ecuador for three years. I had the privilege of sharing in the traditions of other families, many of which were new to me. I also became a vegetarian, so the foods I chose were very different.

I have come to understand that the holidays are times we get to make up for ourselves. Their meaning and significance come from deep within, not from expectations or the superficial goings on around us. Each year I choose old and new activities that remind me of the significance of the season.

And then there is the holiday food. It is so easy to overdo. Almost all of us eat things we normally do not eat at other times of the year. I won't bore you with the statistics about the average weight gain during November and December each year.

My gift to you is a recipe I developed and have enjoyed over the years. I look forward to the holidays when all the ingredients are available. This dish is healthy, delicious, and healing. The acidity of the cranberry has been shown to have a positive effect on the environment of the kidney. It is just about the only recipe I have ever seen for cranberries that doesn't call for lots of sugar. Yes, it can be tart, depending on the type of apples and how many raisins you use. I have always received rave reviews when I take it to a potluck dinner or serve it to guests in my home. It has become one of my personal holiday traditions. I hope you will enjoy it as much as my family and I do.

Homemade Cran-Apple-Raisin Sauce from the Kitchen of Rita Miller-Huey

Makes 8 servings. Takes about 1 hour to prepare.

6 cups apples
12 oz. cranberries (one bag)
½ cup raisins
2 whole cinnamon sticks
⅛ to ¼ cup water
1 cup nonfat vanilla yogurt

1. Clean, core, and cut apples into chunks. Do not peel them.

2. Rinse cranberries, picking out the bad ones.

3. Combine apples, cranberries, and raisins in medium saucepan.

4. Break the cinnamon sticks in two and push into the fruit mixture.

5. Pour the water over the top.

6. Cook over medium-low heat, uncovered, at least 30 minutes until the apples are cooked down to sauce and the cranberries pop. Stir occasionally (it will be chunky).

7. Serve warm or chilled with nonfat vanilla yogurt.

This is a naturally sweet combination because of the raisins. For sweeter sauce, use Rome or Jonathan apples (Red Delicious apples are not good for cooking). For tart sauce, use Macintosh or Granny Smith apples. A combination creates a more complex flavor. Rome and Macintosh are my favorites.

The sauce can be stored up to 2 weeks in the refrigerator; longer in the freezer. Fresh cranberries are only available in November and December, so buy extra bags and freeze them to make this sauce for the 4th of July!

Nutrition analysis per serving: Calories: 115; Fat (g): 0.5; Cholesterol (mg): 0; Protein (g): 1.4; Carbohydrates (g): 28; Fiber (g): 5.

— Rita Miller-Huey, M.Ed., R.D., L.D.

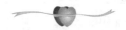

A Recipe for a Special Day for a Special Someone

"Valentine—a person singled out as one's sweetheart on Saint Valentine's Day; A greeting card or gift given on this day" *(Webster's New World Dictionary).*

Why have holidays? To give us an extra reason to make a fuss over the ones we love! As caregivers, we show our love in many ways every day. Yet those everyday things can be minimized in the face of our loved ones' needs. So, for Valentine's Day, do something special to show your loved ones just how much you do love them—not because they need you, but because you wouldn't have it any other way.

Make the day special in a personal way. Take a walk down memory lane. Does your loved one have a story about a special Valentine? When courting? Proposing? A husband or wife? Old beau or girlfriend? Grandchild? What can you do that would remind him or her of that special time? What did your loved one do for his or her Valentine? Can you spark a memory for him or her in some small way? Was it a special food? A special type of candy? A song? A place? An activity?

What is the easiest way you can bring a Valentine to your loved one? Do you have his or her song on a tape or CD? Do you have pictures of "way back when" that you could look at together? Can you listen to your loved one's story just one more time? Could you arrange for a call or visit from a special person? Maybe a videotape? Would fresh flowers or a plant be a treat? Maybe a soft stuffed animal?

Perhaps you could serve a favorite meal in a special way. Dinner by candlelight with votive candles in glass holders, music, a bud vase with a single rose or carnation, a red napkin, a favorite dessert, regardless of diet restrictions.

Giving a Valentine can be fun, too. Together, you can make simple Valentines with lace doilies, construction paper, glue, and magic markers, then mail or deliver them to special people. Some cookies, either homemade or store-bought, but hand-decorated with the frosting in the tube, are fun to do, to give—and receive!

As incessant as caregiving can seem at times, making one day special among many can bring warmth and delight— and a break in what can otherwise be monotonous for all those involved.

— Rita Miller-Huey, M.Ed., R.D., L.D.

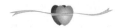

Surviving the Holidays

Holidays and special occasions can bring out the best and worst in us. The prospect of wonderful, happy times abound, filling us with somewhat unrealistic hopes for our relationships. We are often disappointed by how these special occasions turn out. Add to the normal tensions of holidays the image of someone you love being ill or incapacitated, and you have the makings of a very difficult time. Many times we wish we could just disappear until the holidays are over.

Caregivers may have unusually high expectations during holidays and special occasions. Knowing that this might be a last birthday, anniversary, Thanksgiving, Christmas, etc., caregivers may feel enormous pressure to make this time especially significant. The caregiving family faces the normal tensions families experience during the holiday season, but their resources are usually depleted, energy levels are low, and free time is limited.

Some thought and careful planning can make these times easier. First and foremost, we need to try to think about what we really want to happen. Do you want to have a quiet day? Is it important to have anyone in particular around you? If you are a caregiver, you might ask yourself, "What am I up to doing?" Honor your answer by not doing more than you are comfortable doing.

If you choose to have company, make it easy. Don't assume all the responsibility. Ask your loved one what he or she feels up to. Most people usually like to have those they love, and feel comfortable around, with them. Limit these occasions to family members and a few close friends.

Encourage honest communication among the entire family, including close friends. Although your loved one may not seem to know exactly what is going on, try to remember that most care recipients have a real sense about themselves, their illness, and what is going on in their world. Don't allow the person's illness to replace his or her identity. Families can share their sadness and disappointments by talking about them openly. You do not need to force cheerfulness, but don't forget that humor makes many of life's difficulties easier to bear.

Keeping your level of expectations realistic will make the day go smoother for you, your loved one, extended family, and friends. Remember that whatever you choose to do this year does not need to be the same as the past, or the same in the future. If sandwiches on paper plates served in the bedroom are all that is possible, don't try to cook up a turkey dinner.

The best advice for caregivers is: be realistic. Expect the normal tensions of family togetherness. Let others know how they can make the holidays easier for you.

Don't overdo it. Recognize that you may be physically and emotionally depleted. Try to read, exercise, eat well, and get some time alone. Try to stay in the here and now; anticipation is always worse than the actual event. Let yourself dispense with the institutional nature of the holidays and look for ways to make the day meaningful for you and your loved ones.

— Jennifer Kay, L.C.S.W.

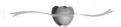

Escaping the Holiday Coulda, Woulda, Shouldas

Enjoying the holidays as a caregiver includes letting go of a dangerous mind-set called coulda, woulda, shoulda thinking, also known as the "if only" syndrome. If there were such a thing as Caregivers Anonymous, the first step to combat this way of thinking would be to rid ourselves of that little voice inside us caregivers that says, "I can do it all. I am responsible for everything. Whatever I do, it's never enough. I coulda, woulda, shoulda . . ."

Here are some ways to ease caregiver stress and ditch the if-only syndrome:

- When planning holiday events, ask guests to come over rather than taking your loved one out. Celebrating at home means your loved one can enjoy the event in a familiar and comfortable setting. He or she can leave the room without breaking up the party.

- Potluck celebrations, with each guest bringing a course, reduces undue stress on caregivers. If it's a casual gathering, you can ask guests to help prepare or even help clean up. If you don't feel comfortable having a potluck party, simply ask guests to bring wine or dessert to ease some of the workload and expense.

- Inviting people over for a meal during your loved one's regular mealtime helps. If you decide to cook dinner yourself, make something that is easily prepared in advance, such as lasagna or stew. Make something on the grill, buy prepared food, or order in. Remember, paper and plastic make cleanup much easier.

- Sometimes your loved one will not join in the holiday celebration. A frail parent may no longer enjoy staying up to greet the New Year. Staying at home with a companion or sitter may be more enjoyable than being dragged into a social situation that may be too tiring or uncomfortable. You can attend holiday events without your loved one. This may also help you refuel. You can't refuel without some distance. Of course, while away, you need to be away completely—mentally and physically.

It's not easy to stop wishing for things that can't be, or regretting what is and daydreaming of how holidays used to be. But learning to clear our minds of this toxic mind-set, even briefly, helps to regain balance and energy. Letting go of hopeless crusades to try to make things how they coulda, woulda, shoulda been is an enormous accomplishment that allows you, and your loved one, to live within the current situation. As they say in those twelve-step programs, we need to acknowledge our limitations and enjoy the here and now.

— Sherry Issa, M.S.W., L.C.S.W., D.A.B.C.M.

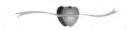

Chapter 10

When In-Home Caregiving Is No Longer Enough

When in-home caregiving becomes more than you or your family can handle, when your loved one's condition demands more professional help, here are some things to consider.

Geriatric Care Managers

As a caregiver you know that prolonged illness, disability, or simply the challenges of aging can significantly alter the lifestyle of older adults. Daily responsibilities can become difficult.

As an adult, balancing work, children, and elder care can be a challenge. It is also a challenge for the older adult whose spouse requires care, and whose own health may be failing. One solution is to hire a professional geriatric care manager (GCM), a professional who specializes in assisting older people and their families facing elder care concerns. They assist older adults in maintaining their independence at home and can ease the transition to a new setting, if needed.

A good GCM takes the time to get to know you and understand your concerns, needs, and wants. Professional GCMs offer a variety of services, including assessment and development of a customized plan of care. They also may implement and monitor the plan whether in the home, a residential care unit, or skilled nursing environment. GCMs have a minimum of a bachelor's degree or higher and training in gerontology, social work, nursing, counseling, psychology, or a related field.

Don't fall prey to inept, overpriced, or unethical GCMs. According to Vicki Zoot, a consultant for CNA Insurance Cos., "It is a big consumer issue. Anybody can hang out a shingle and call themselves a care manager."

How do you find a good GCM? Ask for credentials. Where did he attend school? What is her level of education? How much experience has he had working with older adults? Request references; a good GCM has many.

Do GCMs specialize? Some specialize in working with the memory-impaired or solving complicated problems related to finances, to name just a couple. Does the GCM have liability insurance?

What are the fees? In some states, the hourly fee can range from $50 to $110. At these rates, GCM fees can mount fast. Stay in close contact with the GCM, particularly if you are being charged by the hour, or until a solid relationship is built.

Ask if the GCM has any personal financial interest in referrals that he or she makes. If yes, it may mean that the GCM is referring clients to a particular source because he or she receives a kickback, and not because it is in your best interest.

How does the GCM charge? By the hour or the job? Are you charged for long distance phone calls or driving time?

Most GCMs offer a variety of package rates. Discuss these beforehand to determine what is best for you.

Contact the National Association of Professional Geriatric Care Managers for referrals. Members subscribe to rigorous ethics and standards, and the profession is moving rapidly to set rigid standards. The National Academy of Certified Care Managers offers certification exams. Contact the organization to find out whether your GCM is certified.

— Terry Weaver, M.P.S., N.H.A., C.M.C., A.C.C.

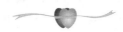

Caregiver-Friendly Facilities

One of my great joys is helping other caregivers avoid some of the pitfalls I encountered when I began my role as caregiver in 1990. Please understand, there are still many challenges to caring for my father. As I'm sure you've discovered with the loved one you care for, just when you think you have one problem solved, another pops up. Your loved one's condition changes, many times for the worse. The financial situation worsens, his or her health deteriorates, and care becomes more difficult. Sometimes, all three happen at the same time.

This is when you might be considering putting your loved one into an assisted living or nursing home facility. If so, you really need what we at *Today's Caregiver Magazine* call a "Caregiver-Friendly Facility," one for which you can answer yes to all of the following questions:

Yes	No	
❑	❑	Are the visiting hours acceptable?
❑	❑	Is there an area where family members can meet with their loved ones?
❑	❑	Are the rooms clean and tidy?
❑	❑	Does the management understand that at least one family member is directly involved in the care of the resident?
❑	❑	Are the staff members honest and open in their communications with the caregiver?
❑	❑	Is the ratio of staff to residents appropriate?
❑	❑	Can a family member find involved and caring staff when he or she goes to the facility— whenever he or she goes there?
❑	❑	Does the facility regularly pass the smell test?
❑	❑	Is the medical staff appropriate for the facility?
❑	❑	Is management interested in your opinion, or are families considered to be a necessary nuisance?
❑	❑	Does management accept your role as advocate, or are you shut out of decisions regarding your loved one?

As you can see, a caregiver-friendly facility is essential, not only for the patient, but for his or her caregiver as well. Caregiver-friendly facilities give you, the caregiver, another pair of watchful eyes, another advocate for your loved one, and another caring soul who wants to give good care to your loved one and maintain the excellence the facility strives for. And if these are things the facility in question does not appreciate, move on. You will be happier, and so will your loved one.

— Monica Weiss Barg

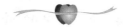

What to Look for in a Nursing Home

Here is a more detailed checklist for assessing nursing homes. If possible, both the caregiver and care recipient should be involved in the decision-making process. The more the patient participates in the planning process, the easier it will be to adjust to the new environment.

The Facility

Yes	No	
❏	❏	Are there handrails along the walls?
❏	❏	Are the doorways wheelchair-accessible?
❏	❏	Does management take safety precautions to prevent residents from falling down the stairs?
❏	❏	Is the floor kept dry and free of litter?
❏	❏	In case of fire, can the facility be evacuated easily?
❏	❏	Are fire extinguishers easy to locate?

Yes	No	
❏	❏	Does the facility appear clean?
❏	❏	Are there lingering odors?
❏	❏	Do the faucets, call buttons, telephones, and television sets work?
❏	❏	Are heating and cooling adequate?

Staff and Care

❏	❏	Is the atmosphere pleasant?
❏	❏	Do staff genuinely seem to enjoy working with the residents?
❏	❏	Do staff appear to care about and respect residents?
❏	❏	Are residents treated as individuals?
❏	❏	Do staff appear interested in the residents?
❏	❏	Do staff seem interested in speaking to visitors or residents?
❏	❏	Are your questions answered clearly, frankly, and in sufficient depth?
❏	❏	Do any other residents have conditions similar to your loved one's?
❏	❏	Are residents clean and adequately dressed?
❏	❏	Do staff appear to refrain from making unrealistic promises or predictions?
❏	❏	Are the rights of the residents posted?
❏	❏	Is the food hot, attractive, and tasty?
❏	❏	Are special diets available? What kinds?

Yes   No

☐   ☐   Do residents have plenty of drinking water easily available?

☐   ☐   Are planned, posted, and varied recreational and social activities available?

☐   ☐   Do the listed activities seem interesting and appropriate?

☐   ☐   Do most of the people at an activity program seem to be participating?

☐   ☐   Are religious services held weekly?

Administration

☐   ☐   Is the facility in good standing with state inspectors?

☐   ☐   Are fees competitive?

☐   ☐   Have fees increased significantly in the past few years?

☐   ☐   Is the fee structure easy to understand and reasonable?

☐   ☐   Does the institution readily reveal what services are covered in the quoted fee and what services are extra?

☐   ☐   Is Medicaid accepted? Is Medicare accepted?

☐   ☐   Are billing and accounting procedures understandable and acceptable?

☐   ☐   Is transportation of patients provided?

☐   ☐   Does a resident advisory council exist?

☐   ☐   Are visiting hours reasonable?

Yes	No	
❏	❏	Are therapeutic services available (speech, physical, and occupational)?
❏	❏	Are social work or other mental health services available?
❏	❏	Are community organizations (library, church group, volunteers) involved?
❏	❏	Do the charge nurses, social workers, department heads, and top-level administrators have geriatric experience and/or education?

Assisted Living Communities

Use the following checklist to assist you in evaluating assisted living communities. If possible, both the caregiver and care recipient should be involved in the decision-making process.

The Facility

❏	❏	As you arrive at the residence, do you like its location and outward appearance?
❏	❏	As you enter the lobby and tour the residence, is the decor attractive and homelike?
❏	❏	Did you and the potential resident receive a warm greeting from staff welcoming you to the residence?
❏	❏	Does the administrator/staff call residents by name and interact warmly with them as you tour the residence?
❏	❏	Do residents socialize with each other and appear to be happy and comfortable?

Yes **No**

❏ ❏ Are you able to talk with residents about how they like the residence and staff?

❏ ❏ Do the residents seem to be appropriate housemates for your loved one?

❏ ❏ Are staff dressed appropriately, personable, and outgoing?

❏ ❏ Are staff members you pass during your tour friendly to you?

❏ ❏ Are visits with the resident welcome at any time?

❏ ❏ Is the community well-designed for residents' needs?

❏ ❏ Are the recreational and nonliving spaces free from storage items or other obstacles?

❏ ❏ Is the floor plan easy to follow?

❏ ❏ Do doorways, hallways, and rooms accommodate wheelchairs and walkers?

❏ ❏ Are elevators available for those unable to use stairways?

❏ ❏ Are handrails available to aid in walking?

❏ ❏ Are cupboards and shelves easy to reach?

❏ ❏ Are floors made of a nonskid material and carpets firm to ease walking?

❏ ❏ Does the residence have good natural and artificial lighting?

❏ ❏ Is the residence clean, free of odors, and appropriately heated/cooled?

Yes **No**

❏ ❏ Does the residence meet local and/or state licensing requirements?

Needs Assessments, Contracts, Costs, and Finances

❏ ❏ Is there a written plan for the care of each resident?

❏ ❏ How long after admission is this care plan written?

❏ ❏ Are the family and resident involved in writing the care plan?

❏ ❏ What is the procedure for assessing a potential resident's need for services, and are those needs reassessed periodically?

❏ ❏ Can a resident be discharged for refusing to comply with a care plan?

❏ ❏ When may a contract be terminated, and what are the facility's refund policies?

❏ ❏ Are there any government, private, or corporate programs available to help cover the cost of services to the resident?

❏ ❏ Is a contractual agreement available to include accommodations, personal care, health care, and supportive services?

❏ ❏ Are additional services available if the resident's needs change?

❏ ❏ Are there different costs for various levels or categories of services?

Other Financial Questions

Yes **No**

❑ ❑ How will you pay for additional services such as nursing care when needed on a temporary basis?

❑ ❑ What are the facility's billing, payment, and credit policies?

❑ ❑ Can residents handle their own finances with staff assistance if they are able to, or should a family member or outside party be designated to do so?

❑ ❑ What is the policy on insurance and personal property?

❑ ❑ Are staff available to meet scheduled and unscheduled needs?

Medication and General Health Care

❑ ❑ What is the residence policy regarding storing medication, assisting with medications, training and supervision of staff, and record keeping?

❑ ❑ Is self-administration of medication allowed?

❑ ❑ Who coordinates home care visits from a nurse, physical therapist, occupational therapist, etc., if needed?

❑ ❑ Are staff available to assist residents who experience memory, orientation, or judgment losses?

❑ ❑ Does a physician or nurse visit residents regularly to provide medical checkups?

❑ ❑ What is the procedure for responding to residents' medical emergencies?

Services

Yes   **No**

☐   ☐   Are staff available to provide twenty-four-hour assistance with activities of daily living (ADL) if needed? ADLs include:

- ☐ Dressing
- ☐ Eating
- ☐ Mobility
- ☐ Hygiene and grooming
- ☐ Bathing
- ☐ Toileting
- ☐ Incontinence
- ☐ Using the telephone
- ☐ Laundry
- ☐ Housekeeping in unit
- ☐ Transportation to doctor, hairdresser, activities, etc.
- ☐ Shopping
- ☐ Walking/caring for pets
- ☐ Others

Features of Individual Units

☐   ☐   Are different sizes and types of units available?

☐   ☐   Are units for single and double occupancy available?

☐   ☐   Do residents have their own lockable doors?

☐   ☐   Is a twenty-four-hour emergency response system accessible from the unit?

Yes   No

❏   ❏   Are bathrooms private and can they accommodate wheelchairs and walkers?

❏   ❏   Are residents able to bring their own furnishings for their unit, and what are they allowed to bring?

❏   ❏   Do all units have a telephone and cable TV, and how is billing handled?

❏   ❏   Is a kitchen area/unit provided with a refrigerator, sink, and cooking element?

❏   ❏   Are residents allowed to keep food in their units?

❏   ❏   Are residents allowed to smoke in their units? In public spaces?

❏   ❏   Are residents allowed to have pets?

Social and Recreational Activities

❏   ❏   Is there evidence of an organized activities program, such as a posted daily schedule, events in progress, reading materials, visitors, etc.?

❏   ❏   Do residents participate in the neighboring community?

❏   ❏   Do volunteers, including family members, come into the residence to help with or conduct programs?

❏   ❏   Does the facility require residents to undertake any chores or perform specific activities that benefit all residents?

Yes   No

☐   ☐   Does the residence have its own pets or provide for pets to visit the facility?

Food Service

☐   ☐   Does the residence provide three nutritionally balanced meals a day, seven days a week?

☐   ☐   Are snacks available?

☐   ☐   Are residents allowed to request special foods?

☐   ☐   Are common dining areas available?

☐   ☐   Are residents allowed to eat meals in their units?

☐   ☐   May meals be provided when residents want them, or are there set times for meals?

— As provided by *Senior Alternatives,* a guide to senior living, (800) 350-0770

The Eden Alternative

— An Interview with Dr. Bill Thomas

Dr. Bill Thomas, a physician with special interest in aging and the elderly, travels around the country encouraging institutional care facilities to adopt his concept, the Eden Alternative, which promotes attending to the emotional and spiritual needs of the elderly with companion animals, plants, gardens, and children. A father of five, Dr. Thomas has written several books dealing with the Eden Alternative philosophy and has received numerous awards for his work.

Gary Barg: How did you become involved in caring for the needs of the elderly, specifically in long-term care facilities?

Dr. Bill Thomas: I trained and prepared myself to become a family doctor and an emergency room physician, and I would have never thought I'd be in long-term care in any way. It was just by chance that I took a part-time job in a nursing home and it sort of exposed me to the work of caring for older people. Here's what I saw right away: simply providing people with appropriate care was not the be-all and end-all. In other words, appropriate treatment for older people was not sufficient. There was a whole other dimension to taking care of people that I thought was not getting adequate attention. In the years that followed, I have really come to know this as a spiritual dimension of caregiving. The fact is, you are taking care of someone who is something more than eighty-seven years old with diabetes and peripheral vascular disease. You are taking care of a distinct, wonderful, unique human being, who never existed before and will never exist again, and there is a need to honor that.

GB: Do you think that sense of honor is missing in most long-term care facilities?

BT: As you know, in institutional forms of long-term care, that is often lost. I began to really reflect on why people find nursing homes, in particular, so abhorrent. I realized that it was not just this sense that people were not going to get their medicine, food, or bath, it is the loss of self. That you stop being "Joe from Mulberry Street" and you become "Mr. Smith in Room

304." People in long-term care have become the sum total of their diagnosis.

I began to ask myself, "What can I do about this?" At first it seemed like not much, but then I realized the secret to improving the quality of life for older people in all kinds of care settings is to create a rich and rewarding environment. It ought to be more like a natural environment and rich in terms of social and biological diversity and less like a cold and bureaucratic institution.

Our elders are plagued by loneliness, helplessness, and boredom, and if we attend carefully to these three plagues, we will do a lot to change the fundamental nature of the care we provide.

GB: What is Eden Alternative?

BT: Eden Alternative is about a new philosophy for caring for frail and disabled people that recognizes the importance of connectedness and interconnectedness in any human life. No matter how demented, frail, or disabled one may be, recognizing that interconnectedness leads us down a wonderful and exciting pathway that is not available to us when we are thinking mechanically or medically.

GB: How does it manifest itself in the Eden Alternative approach to long-term care?

BT: What we do is provide an "Edenizing environment" with companion animals to answer the cry of pain from loneliness. People are encouraged to fall in love with these companion animals, and that is distinctly different from pet therapy, which has its own virtues and uses. I'm talking about an attempt to create bonds of companionship that endure, and for people to invest emotionally in relationships with these animals.

Second, in an Edenizing environment, people help the elderly become caregivers, as well as receivers of care. We find that when older people, especially those with chronic illnesses, care for other living creatures, it improves and is important in maintaining their well-being and self-worth.

Third, in an Edenizing environment, we struggle to create variety and spontaneity. Most institutions care for people on a strict timetable. We try to inject unexpected happenings into daily life by bringing huge numbers of companion animals, plants, and children into the environment.

GB: Is there a particular format that you look for facilities to follow?

BT: We have decided we want every single facility to look and feel different. What we do insist on is that all people commit themselves to the struggle against loneliness, helplessness, and boredom, and that ties each facility together.

GB: How do you get around concerns about the animals running loose and hurting the residents?

BT: First and frankly, the level of dissatisfaction within institutional long-term care is so high that people are willing to kind of stand up and say, "Gosh, let's just try it!" It is pretty hard to argue that everything is fine just the way it is. Number one: this gives us a lot of freedom to try new things because expectations are low.

Number two: by adopting the Eden Alternative, the facility is going to be a lot less like a health care facility. Some staff members, family members, and residents will have a problem with this because they want to maintain the status quo, and this challenges the status quo.

Number three: we conducted observational studies that have shown no negative correlation in terms of accidents, infections, or falls in the Edenizing environment. In fact, there is clearly documented evidence that there is a decrease in the number of infections and medications, especially psychoactive medications for aggressive behavior. The real negative is how difficult it is getting people to change their minds.

GB: Do you mean getting the professionals or families to change their minds?

BT: The families can see what is going on and want some kind of change. The professionals are the difficult ones to change and, being a professional, I have sympathy for them. They are highly regulated and poorly compensated and their institutions have a terrible public reputation. The professionals feel that nothing can be done, and that pervasive sense of defeatism is the biggest drawback.

GB: What have you found to the contrary?

BT: If I have an audience of professionals, I remind them that the health care field is a spiritual calling. Caregiving matters to your heart and soul, so let's start acting like it. When we put some of these spiritual dimensions at the heart of our work, we make a better environment for the care recipient and ourselves. The opening of their hearts will open their minds to some of the difficult and strange ideas we have to offer as part of the Eden Alternative.

GB: **How does this approach help caregivers? How have you seen it affect them?**

BT: The number one rule that we spend time teaching people is: as management does unto the caregiver, so shall the caregiver do unto the elder. If management creates a punitive and bureaucratic work environment for professional caregivers, then they re-create that very same environment for the elders.

In terms of the family caregiver and the care facility, we find there is an exclusion of the family caregiver. For example, here I have Mrs. Jones who, for sixty-five years, has been the wife, the partner, the caregiver, and sustainer of Mr. Jones. On June 2, he is admitted to a nursing home. On June 2, Mrs. Jones becomes a "visitor," with no power and a lot of fear. Mrs. Jones is taken out of her role as caregiver and is strongly discouraged from any ongoing caregiving relationship with her husband.

What Eden does is create something we call the middle ground. We create an environment rich with children, plants, and animals, and that same Mrs. Jones becomes the caregiver for the environment. You must sustain caregiving, even in the context of an institutional arrangement. Along that same line, from the Eden philosophy, we say move decision-making authority back to the elders, and if there is a decision the elders cannot make, the decision goes to the people who are closest to the elders.

GB: What can caregivers do to promote their facility's interest?

BT: Left to its own devices, the long-term care industry is not going to change. Family caregivers need to put themselves in front of the administrator in their office with the door closed and say, "It can be different." Ultimately, that will be the force that changes long-term care.

There is no administrator in America who does not know about the Eden Alternative. There are some administrators who will argue that they don't have the time to get mixed up with all those dogs and cats, and they are the ones who are missing out. It is not about dogs and cats; it is about creating an environment centered on spiritual and human growth that includes the staff, family members, and elders. It is putting aside the medical model and searching instead for a more human model of how we take care of the elderly.

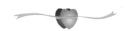

Chapter 11

And in the End

And in the end, the love you take
is equal to the love you make.
— Paul McCartney

Losses

Given a choice, I would hold fast to you—
  would stop the slow erosion of our lives.
It isn't fair that we who've loved so long
  should be the losers, even though we love.
We are not what we were, nor will we be
  the travelers of our dreams, and journey far.
We try to hold the edges of our lives
  and yet they slip away, out of our grasp
Like sands the waves consume along the shore.
The edges crumble, but the center holds—
  you are still you, and I am still myself.
That will not change. The loving will endure,
  through illness, age, and death (the final loss).
I cling to what we have, and push away
  the thought of how, by inches, as I watch
You seem somehow diminished, letting go
  of little daily things you cannot hold.

We walk this path together, after all,
    and if you stumble, I will take your hand,
And if I tremble, you will hold me tight.
    All is not lost to the approaching night.

— Camilla Hewson Flinterman

"Okay, We Go Now."

That phrase always signaled a decisive end of my grandfather's visit to my parent's house when I was younger. With those words, my grandfather would rise abruptly from the couch, sneak dollar bills into my hands and the hands of my siblings, and drive off, more often than not in the paint-encrusted white Chevrolet station wagon he used in his work as a painting contractor.

A decidedly handsome man, he reminded everyone of a Hungarian Cesar Romero with dark, thick, wavy hair, which in later years turned shock-white, all the while maintaining its thick texture. I can still sense his smells—the aftershave mingled with the lingering scent of lacquer and paint thinner, whichever he had used last.

His strong, sure hands were those of a true artisan, chiseled and firm as only a man who has used them in labor for decades would possess, yet at the same time gentle, passionate, and artistic. The hands one would imagine a painter on the left bank of Paris would gesture with to judge the scope and shape of a scene about to be painted. My grandfather would wave those hands before any scene as if he were able to transpose the images directly onto canvas through thin air.

This was a man of great contradictions, wearing jackets mismatched to pants, but always jacketed and always elegant.

Until his very last days, he would never hesitate to kiss any woman's hand when she entered his room. He was strong, firm, and direct, but a kidder of the first degree.

One of my most favorite (and conversely, one of my younger brother's least favorite) memories is of a fishing trip the three of us took many years ago. I couldn't have been older than twelve, and my brother eight years old. We went on a chartered deep-sea fishing boat out of Miami, Florida.

The boat was filled with other families seeking marlin, tarpon, or yahoo, but more likely than not were just catching colds, good memories, and deep sunburns (these were, after all, the sixties, and the idea that a sunburn could cause skin cancer into the next millenium had not even been imagined).

The weather was particularly nasty, and as the boat heaved across the turbulent seas, my brother was experiencing his own heaving down below. Owing as much to his bad luck that day, the head (or bathroom), where he spent the bulk of that trip, was located right next to the dining table where my grandfather and I were consuming great quantities of the fried chicken, potato salad, and pickles packed with loving care by my grandmother. Suffice it to say that the timing of our turning to the bathroom door and crunching pickles or devouring chicken drumsticks was coincidental with my brother's brief but colorful visits outside the bathroom door. He was as green as the ocean and the color of the ship. As I said, a great memory.

My grandfather came to this country in the 1930s, yet he never lost his thick and luxurious Romanian accent. Born in Transylvania, the land of Dracula and shifting borders, he jumped ship into the waters of the Baltimore harbor off a Russian freighter onto which he had been consigned at the age of seventeen. Making his way to New Jersey, he became an American citizen, and at the age of thirty-five, he enlisted to fight in World War II. He became a baker in the Navy construction forces (the Seabees). This, according to my mother, was a mixed blessing, because after the war, he could never seem to be able to adapt the army recipes designed for battalions to baking for his family of three. My mom fondly remembers giving away or throwing out mountains of extra cake and cookies whenever he took to the kitchen.

Another brother story: When my brother was in his late teens and enrolled in Miami Dade Community College, among his classmates was (you guessed it) my grandfather. Desiring to complete his interrupted education, my grandfather enrolled in courses at the same college. I have to admit that seeing your grandfather on the dean's list semester after semester could certainly be disconcerting to any college student!

I returned home for a visit to celebrate my grandfather's eightieth birthday celebration in 1987. As I entered my mother's house, I saw my grandfather standing on a chair that was placed on top of a desk in my childhood bedroom. He was painting the house. The entire house. Alone. Why? "Because it should look good for the celebration." And besides, he had been meaning to do it for a while.

In the mid-nineties, when in his mid-eighties, my grandfather started showing signs of early-stage Alzheimer's. This was a devastating blow to the entire family. Here was invincible Joe Weiss, the man who, until his seventies, had never been a patient in any hospital, who worked until his early eighties, and who was, in the truest sense, adored by his extended family.

Our goal from that point forward was to create a sense of what I call *transparent caregiving*. We would construct a world where he felt he was still in charge, but where he was also safe from harm. The adult day care center where he spent the day became "his job." He would stand outside his apartment complex and wait for the bus to take him "to work." During off days, he would be "on vacation." Monica Dunkley, a magnificent caregiver who ran the center, took him under her wing. But to Gramp, his boss was the male activities director. In Gramp's time, the bosses were usually men, so this man was boss. Which was fine with everyone concerned, including Monica.

In time, as my grandfather's disease progressed, the day came where adult day care was no longer an appropriate answer, and, when his medical needs changed, he moved from assisted living to nursing home care. Throughout the entire time, though, he never failed to brighten up when my mom, his daughter, entered the room. She was the center of his universe and was always there for him.

I loved to sit for long periods holding his hand and "talking" with him, about what, I will never know. I will always remember these as bittersweet moments; on one hand, I savor the times we spent together and cherish the occasions he would smile and point to his mouth, asking for a kiss, which I administered cheerfully. On the other hand, I have never felt sadder for him. Sometimes while in the assisted living facility, he would hit his head repeatedly, as if to say, "I know I am not thinking as well as I should and I am no longer in control." As if he could beat his mind to be better, like hitting the side of a soda machine when the drink fails to appear. Although I could always redirect his energies and he eventually stopped the practice, this fleeting acknowledgment of his own failing mind haunts me to this day.

The day he died, I was packed and ready to travel to New York for business. It was about 9:45 in the morning and, as I sat on the couch in my apartment, I suddenly looked over my shoulder at a picture on the wall behind me. It was a self-portrait Gramp had painted in the mid-seventies. The face that he saw looking back at him when he painted this portrait was strong and kind and handsome, with no idea of what lay ahead. A moment in time came alive for me at that instant, and that image replaced the face afflicted by advanced age and illness, the one I had become used to over these past few years.

At 10:00, as I left the house and got into the car to go to the airport, I received a call from my brother, at the hospital where our grandfather had been battling pneumonia for the past week. Gramp was gone. He had passed about fifteen minutes earlier.

To this day, when thinking of Gramp, I can only conjure up the self-portrait, painted so many years ago, which hangs over my couch. Not his later visage. One last gift from Gramp.

"Okay. We go now."

— Gary Barg

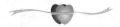

Family Care List

The most loving gift you can give your family is to put your affairs in order before a disaster or medical emergency strikes. To assist in providing that gift, here is a list of the information and documents you should have prepared.

- All bank accounts, account numbers, and types of accounts and the location of bank
- Insurance company, policy numbers, beneficiary as stated on the policies, and type of insurance (health, life, long-term care, automobile, etc.)
- Deeds and titles to *all* property
- Loan/lien information, who holds them, and if there are any death provisions
- Social Security and Medicare numbers
- Military history, affiliations, and papers (including discharge papers)
- Up-to-date will in a safe place (inform family where the will is located)
- Living will or other advance directive appropriate to your state of residence
- Durable power of attorney
- Instructions for funeral services and burial (if arrangements have been secured, name and location of funeral home)

— *Today's Caregiver Magazine*

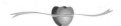

C.A.R.E.

The days may be getting longer, but the hours seem to be shorter in the final days of your caregiving. Things are happening so fast that you can't seem to put your finger on any one thing before it changes again. How do you make the final days more comfortable and right for your mother, father, child, or anyone else for whom you have cared?

Do you need a full- or part-time nurse? Do you need a medical institution, such as a nursing home, hospital, or hospice? How do you go about making the decision?

You may have backing from a family member, or even a good friend, but in most cases probably not. The doctor, minister, or rabbi and a knowledgeable attorney should be working with you to help you make the most appropriate decisions. Sometimes it's hard to ask for or even take advice from others when you've been in control for so long. But for your sake, as well as your charge's, relent somewhat and listen. They are professionals and they know better. The professionals think with their knowledge, not just their hearts; absorb and listen. Remember, you still have to make the final decision.

I know it may be a difficult topic to face, but preneed arrangements must be made. The best advice I can offer a caregiver is to *stop,* take a breath, get someone to take charge for a few hours, then do something for yourself, such as thinking of something serene and pleasant and caring, being selfish, listening to soothing music, calling a friend and chatting for a while, writing a funny letter to someone (if only to yourself), going for a walk in the mall or in the park, going to a movie and losing yourself in the story, meeting friends for lunch, going to the library and getting the book you have been wanting to read for a long time, going anywhere you want.

Take in a change of scenery, because this time is medicine for you, the caregiver. Without this you may well wind up as someone else's charge. Look at the beauty of the sun rising in the morning, or the moon and stars at night. Feel yourself floating in the heavens—even though it may be brief. *Do it.*

Remember—the caregiver is also important!

C.A.R.E.

C—COMMITMENT

A—ACTION

R—RESULTS

E—EMPOWERMENT

Commitment is something you have made to a loved one.

Action is what you know has to be taken for a loved one.

Results are what you want for your loved one.

Empowerment is what you receive when you are able to bring together commitment, action, and results for your loved one.

C.A.R.E., as in caregiver, is one of the most important words in any language.

— Monica Weiss Barg

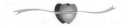

Journey East

Whenever we determine to leave our island home and head for the mainland (we live on the slopes of Mauna Loa, an active volcano on the Big Island of Hawaii), a great process is set in motion. Not just the travel arrangements and the things needing attention to make the journey happen, but something more mysterious. We've never journeyed east without this happening.

When I think about it, it is very much like what happens in the Hebrew month of Elul, a time when rabbis gather their strength from deep within. For the Jewish people it is a time of great reflection and preparation. In ancient times the shofar was blown each morning of Elul to awaken all to what would always follow: the first ten days of the month of Tishri, the Jewish High Holy Days, beginning with Rosh Hashanah and ending with Yom Kippur.

The month of Elul is fraught with anticipation and surfacing fears, as are the journeys to hometowns, old friends, and loving or scorned relatives. Both become a time of deep personal questioning, consideration of making amends, and, God willing, a time of healing spiritual and, often, physical wounds.

This past summer I made that journey east, much like the journey from Elul to Tishri. The events of this summer held the beauty of never really knowing an outcome, and the gifts of living with hope and the strength of love.

The journey east was initiated by a cry of desperation on the part of my sister-in-law who has been the sole caregiver to her husband (my husband's brother) and was facing burnout. He has had multiple sclerosis most of his adult life, almost all of their married life. My husband and his brothers, traveling from all parts of the country, were determined to meet in Florida to see if they could resolve the crisis.

You can well imagine the anguish preceding this event, the times of overwhelming and unbearable pain for the family. All of them questioning their true feelings about and commitment to their brother. Weighing responsibility against guilt, obligations against love, inner strength against silent fears. When the brothers met, they agreed that a particular facility they were considering was a surprisingly good alternative, with caring staff who treated their brother with kindness and respect. My sister-in-law is able to take him out several times a week for activities he has always enjoyed, like fishing and bird watching. And, out of this seemingly hopeless situation, the brothers reunited. They had a wonderful time together, swimming with dolphins, watching their brother feeling free in the water, loving and supporting each other as a family. They have determined to continue meeting like this—rekindling their connection, expressing their love.

During this same pilgrimage, we visited my relatives in the north. My cousins were celebrating their anniversary. It was a joyous time. Then suddenly, in the middle of the night, one cousin died of a massive heart attack. It was an incredible shock, no warning signs. He just went to sleep and never woke up. He wasn't ill a day in his life and embodied strength and admiration for all who knew and loved him.

I was asked to do the eulogy, then *shiva* (a week of mourning) began. That was the beginning of the Elul atmosphere for us, as a family. I remember the evening the closest members of the family decided to retreat up in my cousin's room. His pocket change was still out on the side of the bed, his clothes, his widow and children bearing witness to his physical departure. About eighteen of us were there. We talked, wept, and hugged each other.

The mystery began to reveal itself again: the Divine light within us all, the love that binds our souls, the eternal truth that is not physical but ethereal and otherworldly. My husband's brothers connected with it in the hardship they faced, as did my family in its grief and loss. These are the days of awe, all the days of our lives that cannot be erased and that serve to strengthen us in our darkest hours.

May all caregivers and their loved ones know abundant blessings. May they be renewed with courage and strengthened by the healing power of unconditional love.

— Rabbi Rita Leonard

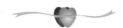

After Caregiving: Picking Up the Pieces

As caregivers, we become totally committed to caring for another person. Our loved one is no longer able to function in the normal routine of life. We move in with our loved one, or he or she moves in with us. We give up our jobs, our own independence, and very often our family and friends. We become so involved with the care of that person that we become removed from normal day-to-day living.

Our entire life revolves around comforting and helping our loved one feel loved. We protect that person at all costs. In a very real sense, we have given our life for another. We do this, not out of obligation, but because of love. The commitment that we make is the ultimate test of love for another.

Then one day we wake up, and our responsibility has ended. Our loved one has been released to a far greater love, has gone to a place of no more pain or suffering. The time has come to face our grief. We must begin the difficult process of finding our way back into the world.

How do we pick up the pieces and start to live again? We all need to follow our own individual path. It comes down to taking one step at a time. Some people can speed their way back out into the world. Some of us walk more slowly than others. Often we find ourselves taking one step forward and two steps back.

Returning to a normal life is not an easy process. As difficult as that transition is, one thing is certain. There *is* a life after caregiving! We just have to look forward and embrace the many opportunities that are out there for us.

We can renew old friendships or find a job that we feel good doing. We can volunteer for a worthy organization. We can find a new hobby or dust off an old one. We must begin to take a few small steps toward living again.

Finding a friend to talk with is one of the best therapies there is. A friend can listen and support you as you ease back into the world. Soon you will find that life does still exist and that you are a part of it. Butterflies fly among the flowers, and birds still sing in the trees. You just need to open up yourself to experience life once more. The light of another day is showing through, and all that you gave up was well worth it in the end.

Your life has been enriched forever by the choice you made to care for a loved one. No one can ever take that total love away as you rejoin the cares and pleasures of the world.

— Brenda Race

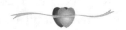

Spaghetti Sandwiches and Banana Popsicles

My grandmother always wore an apron in the kitchen, served sunset-colored Cheez Curls in sunny yellow bowls, maintained a fresh supply of banana popsicles, made the best-tasting miniature pizzas, and nice thick hearty soup and spaghetti sandwiches to keep us giggling.

She was a lady—regal in stature, never too much sun on her delicate rosy cheeks, which contrasted with her fair complexion. Her hair was coal black, even at seventy years old. She always looked nice, even when gardening. Grandma's thumb was kelly green; plants seemed to bend toward her as she moved.

I don't remember the last time I was alone with her while she could still communicate, and I have no idea what we talked about. She always supported my dreams, and I had such plans to share with her. My life would be good, and I would be able to spoil her—buying her whatever dresses she wanted, with shoes and jewelry to match.

When I was a child she was always there for us. If we had a problem, she wanted to know the root, not the surface feelings. Her bosom was always there for comfort and safety when the Wicked Witch from the West appeared on her color TV while we watched *The Wizard of Oz*, eating Cheez Curls from bright yellow bowls. Her smile was sunny. When my brother John and I had the chicken pox, it was Grandma Shaffer who took care of us in isolation while the other four kids stayed at home with Mom and Dad.

Mother's Day, ten years ago, all of us had gathered to celebrate the matrons of our family. As Grandma was leaving the party, she swayed just a bit. I caught her arm until her balance returned. I asked if she was dizzy. She matter-of-factly told me that sometimes she tipped over. When I asked her to see a doctor, she refused. But when I told her that she was too important to us and begged her to see a doctor, she went the next day, Monday. It was her first visit in more than forty years.

On Wednesday she had put both hands to my face, cradling my dimpled cheeks (Grandma's genetic gift to me). She sobbed and looked deeper into my eyes than I ever thought someone could look. She cried. I cried. I promised that we would find out what was wrong and fix it. Hang on, we won't leave you alone. By Friday, she was in a coma. The doctors diagnosed Creutzfeldt-Jakob Disease, a rare and progressive brain virus. I made the eighty-mile round-trip visit to the hospital nearly every day after work, stopping only to visit hospital libraries, searching for information and a cure. All we could find on this disease was not enough to satisfy my need for research and understanding, but there was nothing else.

The doctors could only keep her comfortable. Death was imminent; she was expected to live only a few more weeks. The doctors said she couldn't see or hear us. Still, I couldn't give up hope, however small. Every day I asked her to hang on while we researched to find a cure. Grandma lingered in her coma for more than six months. She was moved from the hospital to a local nursing home, and our visits became less frequent.

We watched her former ladylike stature transform to a fetal position. Her coal black hair was still coal black, but her eyes were distant and empty. We exhausted the research to no avail.

My mother called me early one morning and told me Grandma was going to die that day. Mom wanted to be alone with her. She'd whispered in her ear that we couldn't find a cure; it was all right to go now: we love you and we'll miss you. Mom said the same words that Grandma had said to her mother to let her know it was all right to go: "I will miss your phone calls." Grandma died within a half-hour.

It's not easy letting go, even when you know it's right. I had no idea how much of this experience would stay with me and guide me as I nurtured my career in long-term health care administration. Grandma Shaffer is with me every day, like a beacon to light the way of greater affinity when assisting the caregivers in the facilities in which I work. I miss you Grandma. Thanks for the spaghetti sandwiches and banana popsicles.

— Dan Horter

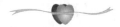

Planning for the Future

Caregivers are lonely people. The more fortunate ones may be surrounded by close family and friends, but many are left to struggle with the pain of a loved one by themselves. My pastoral visits to hospitals and nursing homes introduce me to wives, husbands, and children standing vigil at the bedside of individuals in a game of hide-and-seek with the angel of death. Too often, we remain firm in our conviction that death is the final defeat; it is our enemy. Actually, my faith suggests the hope that death is not an end, merely a transition. It remains one of the last taboos of our culture in which eternal youth and materialism are the measure of our success as persons. Consequently, death is often left as an afterthought.

People do make final arrangements, but these are usually matters of caskets and gravesites, rather than the content of the funeral itself. Usually planning for the future involves legal and financial planning; we consider what we will leave to our children and grandchildren. These issues are too often merely matters of property and money. Yet the very fact of our illness and eventual death is a reminder that what is immortal is not eternal. Matter is temporal; everything is finally fossilized except the human spirit. Indeed, as both individual and caregiver witness the physical container of life deteriorate, it becomes important to focus on the transcendent content of that container—the soul.

The funeral can be a service of healing and transition, a celebration of life and a loved one's sacred and cherished ideals and values. Painfully absent from the final arrangements is consideration and planning for a meaningful and respectful service. In the health care community it appears especially obvious that this aspect of life is often ignored or minimized. Funeral directors ask families whether they belong to a congregation. If the answer is negative, then a clergyman is selected from a list. We are a bit more careful in selecting a lawyer or physician; sometimes one invests more research in choosing a hairdresser.

Caregiving is shepherding. It is accompanying someone on a journey (at least partway). If that journey is to be a good one, then not the pain, the anxiety, or the anticipation of its destination can be trivialized. Illness is a journey on a spiritual plane rather than a topographical one. To be competent shepherds, we must be courageous and loving. We must dare to speak of our fears and sadness; we must discover that our shared spirituality provides other modes of communication. By exploring with our loved ones our feelings about separation and our thoughts about immortality, we establish a meaningful context for this journey whose destination is the final reunion that many traditionalists believe await us.

At the funeral, we realize that pain and anguish are no longer part of our loved one's life. Instead, we turn our attention to how and why that life was lived and what lessons can be derived from our loved one's journey into eternity. The funeral service becomes the last element in caregiving because it demonstrates the manner in which we honor the human spirit as much as we tend to the body that temporarily houses that spirit.

— Rabbi Saul Goldman

Once a Caregiver

What do you do when you're not a caregiver anymore? Are you ever not a caregiver? The matter was brought home to me when my father came to visit. He was the primary caretaker of my stepmother, Rita, who had Alzheimer's for six years.

Telling you how wonderful Rita was would more than fill a magazine by itself, but that's another subject. My father stayed with her at home and barely left her side in all that time. I can't tell you how amazing just that fact alone is to me. Before becoming a caregiver, my father never stayed in one place for ten minutes, let alone for months and years at a time. He was always working or playing hard. He would never stop for a minute. Taking care of Rita turned his life completely around. When she died, all those hours filled with caregiving were suddenly empty and he almost went nuts trying to figure out what he was going to do next.

It took him a while to figure it out. He took walks on the beach. He traveled. He decided to learn how to play golf, which he very much enjoys, but somehow that wasn't enough. He took a job that lasted for a week, I think. He had always been his own boss and working for someone else on a schedule, at a job he didn't really care about, just wasn't going to cut it.

One day he found his way into a long-term care facility and started to play the piano for the residents there. My father has a gift for playing by ear. You hum a tune and he can play it, always could. I don't know what made him decide to do this, but playing for the people there has given him something valuable and meaningful to do. The staff tells him he seems to have an affinity for the people living with Alzheimer's. Imagine that!

At dinner the other night he was telling me about what it means to him to help those people, and that his visits are the highlight of their week. He didn't say it, but I think it is his as well. But why not? He is a caregiver, after all.

— Nancy Schonwalter

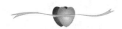

Learning How to Be a Caregiver

It was a beautiful day in March 1995 when my mother and father gathered their family around and my father told us, in his usual intellectual, matter-of-fact way, he was going to die. He talked of living wills, powers of attorney, who would do what and when. How things would be. He cried and we cried. He talked to all of his grandchildren individually.

We spent the day, each of us talking with Dad, alone and together, each of us crying. My father had recurrent fourth-stage melanoma. Untreatable. Incurable. His expected life span was five or six months.

My father was the one who took care of our family. He had been father, friend, mentor, colleague, business associate, therapist, home repair advisor, ad infinitum, to our entire family. Who would take care of me when he was gone? We were losing a true caregiver.

Knowledge did not prepare us, nor could it comfort us. And there was no time for us to get used to the idea, as if that were possible. Throughout my father's valiant attempts at treatment (he endured them all without complaint, knowing they might buy an extra few weeks), he still took care of us all. He stayed in charge. He made all of the necessary appointments and travel arrangements and comforted us in our grief. Even in the last few days of his life, when he could barely speak, he knew my sadness and would pat my check when I cried.

My father's illness was not drawn out for years. It was as if he was fine, and then he wasn't, and then he was gone. I wouldn't be his caregiver in his long twilight years, repaying him for all the times he was there for me. I began to wonder if I could do the job right, if I had the ability, the skills to take care of others the way my father so effortlessly took care of us.

As the cancer wore him down, I realized that he had long ago given me his wonderful life skills to connect with. He taught me to love and have strong, passionate convictions. He taught me how to care for myself: to rest when weary, to take a break when needed. He taught me to sit close and be quiet and how to find the peace of having someone you love nearby.

He taught me to be realistic about death and acknowledge its presence. My father gave me the skills I needed to be there for him, and for my mother, the last week of his life. Long before we ever knew it would be necessary, he taught me how to help him die at home. Without ever noticing the lessons, I had learned how to be a caregiver.

— Jennifer Kay, L.C.S.W.

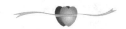

Would I Do It All Over Again?

In a heartbeat I would do it again.
Nothing can take away from me what I did then.
I did the best that I could . . . I gave it my all
And now I can hold up my head . . . and forever
    stand TALL.

I couldn't, I wouldn't change what I did for YOU.
It was done out of LOVE, not out of some due!
If you had stayed here for a thousand years
It would have been worth all of the tears.

You taught me lessons throughout my life,
Ones I used when you were going through the strife.
You showed me well the meaning of LOVE,
Unconditional LOVE that came from above.

You raised me with your love and let me fly free
and then I returned when you needed me.
You continued to teach me when you weren't even
    aware
That the greatest lessons you were yet to share.

For in your dying you gave to me
A compassion that I alone never would see
Had I not taken you under my care,
Giving it my all with nothing to spare.

Would I do it all over again or would I flee?
I would not, could not change it you see.
To LOVE you and comfort you in your time of need
Was not a great task . . . I was only returning the seed.

The seed you planted as you guided me along
Back in the days when YOU were strong!
It was only natural to return the LOVE
Not a chore, but an HONOR, imparted by the one
    above!

— Brenda Race

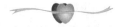

"Let's Not Talk about That Now . . ."

Too often families do not like to talk about issues surrounding death, dying, and funerals. Why should they ask? Soon enough all of us will have to deal with these issues. So what's wrong with waiting until the need arises?

Just like you need to know about health insurance, life insurance, Social Security benefits, and living wills, knowing about funeral arrangements and cemetery property helps you make the financial and emotional decisions you will be comfortable with in years to come.

Over the years, the funeral and cemetery industry has changed. It makes sense for consumers to preplan their arrangements, not only because there is incentive to do so, but even more, because there are also many emotional benefits to prearrangements.

You and your family should consider the following questions:

- What's really involved in a funeral arrangement? Most families, if asked this question will answer, "They pick up the body and take it to the cemetery." Nothing could be further from the truth! A good funeral director will sit with your family and hear what your family members are saying.

- Do you all want the same kind of funeral?

- Do you all agree on the same casket?

- Are there feuding members of the family who will want to be heard at the funeral?

- Who will speak?

- What type of clergy will be appropriate for your family?

- How will your loved one's memory be reflected at the service?

- Will you have a service at all? If not, will you regret it later?

In addition to preparing many documents and obtaining appropriate signatures, arranging for the death certificate to be signed, and notifying Social Security of the death, the funeral director is a liaison among the family, clergy, and cemetery staff. If selected wisely, your funeral director will be your family's advisor, helping each member to feel comfortable and making sure that your wishes are being honored. Funeral directors work behind the scenes from the moment they are contacted, ensuring that things are being done correctly and in a timely manner.

What is involved in purchasing cemetery property? Most cemeteries have many different properties available. You may choose a niche (a space in a mausoleum to place the cremated remains), a grave in a section with a headstone or in a section that has only flat markers, a crypt in a community mausoleum, or a separate, private family mausoleum. There may be a requirement for an outer enclosure (sometimes called a vault) as well as labor fees for burial.

How important is the location? Is convenience for visiting, beauty of the cemetery, or being in or near the family plot the greatest priority? If a cemetery is located in a residential neighborhood, how will you feel as the neighborhood changes? Is this your second marriage, and which spouse would you like to be buried with? Do you want to purchase extra plots for unmarried siblings or children and their families? These are just a few of the issues you need to consider.

What are your family's values about funerals and cemeteries? Often, I hear people saying things like, "Just give me the cheapest funeral possible: I won't be here to know the difference." While this may make economic sense to you, it frequently leaves those behind without a sense of closure. Funerals are a time for people (whether it is two or two hundred) to come together to say good-bye and honor the deceased. It is important for your family to have a dialogue and consider everyone's feelings. In addition, not everyone in a family has the same religious beliefs. These feelings need to be considered as well. Usually almost everyone's needs can be respected if they are discussed in advance.

Remember that prearrangements are a blueprint for your wishes. While funeral or cemetery preneed counselors can help you with these decisions, they cannot anticipate all your family's needs. Therefore, these arrangements are flexible and can be changed. At the time of death, your funeral director will meet with a spokesperson for the family and review all the arrangements to make sure the family information is correct. At that time, adjustments are made if needed. Before you choose a funeral director and cemetery, you might want to take the time to visit the facility and meet the staff with whom you will be working.

Consider whether you have talked with your family about this important topic. While many people feel that their family can take care of this at the time of their death, they do their surviving family no service by leaving it until then. Like any other major purchase you make, you should be an informed consumer and get the information in advance.

— Jennifer Kay, L.C.S.W.

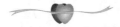

In the Midst of Heroes

The other day on television, I heard a commentator bemoaning the lack of heroes in today's society. He could not have been more wrong. I know because I work in the midst of true heroes. The word *hero* comes from the Greek, meaning to watch over and protect. It is exactly in this context that I, as a home health aide, observe today's heroes. They are the mothers, fathers, sisters, and brothers who have assumed the role of caregiver to the chronically ill and disabled population.

These roles are not sought after, not applied for. There is no time to prepare, and in most instances these roles are permanent. They cause complete role reversals: husbands take on the functions of wives, wives assume the duties of husbands, and children accept responsibility for their parents.

There is a delicate balance, which these heroes maintain: that of assuming a new role in the family, and the care recipients need to be reminded that they are still an integral part of the family. This balancing act necessitates reaching deep within ourselves to find both the physical and emotional strength to deal with it on a daily basis. I have watched the metamorphosis take place. It occurs gradually until the roles are eventually assimilated.

People who have approached problem solving with proactive strategies all their lives now discover themselves not solving problems, but only reacting to each new situation. They find that the ability to adapt has become absolutely necessary because circumstances continue to evolve.

The same people who have helped others all their lives are now in need of assistance, and they do not know how to ask for what they need. Caregivers are unable to leave the house and begin to feel isolated. It becomes imperative that those in the health care industry are sensitive to this and facilitate coping. These ordinary people accomplish extraordinary feats, assuming new roles in the family and finding new ways of coping without sacrificing anyone's humanity.

The responsibility of the individual case manager is overwhelming and frightening, particularly at the onset of home care. I have watched as families somehow reorganize the daily tasks, learn the medical routine, and begin to carve out a new, albeit different, lifestyle. These families are the real heroes and truly one of this country's natural resources.

The same people who have helped others all their lives are now in need of assistance, and they do not know how to ask for what they need.

— Julie A. Koroly

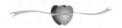

Caregiving: Along Life's Continuum

— An Interview with Cokie Roberts

Cokie Roberts has won numerous awards including the Edward R. Murrow Award and an Emmy. Currently she is Chief Congressional Analyst for ABC News and coanchor with Sam Donaldson of *This Week with Sam Donaldson and Cokie Roberts.* In addition, Ms. Roberts is a news analyst for National Public Radio. She is, and has been for the past seven years, moderator for the Hospice Foundation of America's annual teleconference. She has also been a caregiver to her sister.

Gary Barg: Tell me what your personal interest in Hospice is. Did it come about from your role in caregiving for your sister?

Cokie Roberts: No, but I came to understand how important it is as the positive way of approaching death. I felt very strongly that this was important to talk about and very few people who knew anything about television were able to talk about it. So, they came to me figuring that the combination of the fact that I had cared for someone who was dying and that I could put a television program on the air and, more important, get it off the air, was a good combination. The calls that come in are just unbelievable. And they've done a very good job of not only putting together good people to talk about the different aspects of death and dying over the years, but also the taping throughout the broadcast is so moving. There are times when you'll be sitting there on the set with tears streaming down your cheeks.

GB: **There are so many misunderstandings about Hospice in general, and I know that caregivers still misunderstand Hospice. What in particular would you like to say to help people understand what Hospice really is?**

CR: It's not some dreaded thing. I think there is a sense that if you call in Hospice then you might as well just call the funeral home, and that's not the case. Also, I think that people still really don't understand that you don't have to go to a building called a hospice. They need to understand that (a) Hospice is not going away, it's staying home, and (b) that it can last over a period of months and that it is a service not only for the person who is terminally ill but for the whole family. The family often needs a great deal more help than the person who is sick, not only in terms of care but in dealing with dying. I've found often that the person who is dying can cope with it, that he or she has caught on, and the family is just nowhere near where the person who is dying is.

GB: **You've said that caregiving is a continuum. Can you explain what you mean by that?**

CR: I mean that the message I always try to give to young women is, first of all, don't think—and I do this at women's college graduations all the time—don't think that there is only a certain period of your life where you're a caregiver...When your children are small. When your parents are old, whatever it is. What women do is take care. That's what we do. We do a lot of other stuff, too, but what our mission on this earth is, as far as I'm concerned—and I know I get a lot of argument on it, but that's tough—is taking care. Sometimes it is taking care of the planet or the library or the cultural center or whatever it is, but usually even if that is what a woman's focus is, she's also taking care of human beings, and it's not necessarily just your own children when they're small or when they're having problems along the way or whatever or your own parents.

GB: That's what we tell caregivers all the time. You know, we're asked, "Well, what makes a successful caregiver or a successful caregiving situation?" A lot of it has to do with flexibility and no assumptions of what you expect life to bring you.

CR: Right. It's not fair to have expectations of what life is going to bring you. I mean, life is going to come up and hit you between the eyebrows and say, "Hello." And you know that's one of the great myths. People will say when someone has been sick for a very long time and a spouse has had to really exhaust himself or herself taking care of the person, "Oh, it must be a relief." Well, that's just so stupid. I mean, the truth is it's an enormous hole in your life after you lose somebody that you have been taking care of.

GB: What advice would you give caregivers about that balancing role they need to play?

CR: Well, I think a lot of what we're going to talk about in this teleconference this year is... and I think particularly for the professional caregivers, that you do have to protect yourself.

GB: That's very interesting. I like the way you put that, that you have to protect yourself. I had a reporter ask me the other day if martyrdom was a sign of good caregiving. I said, "Well, martyrdom will get you into anything, but it won't get you out."

CR: You end up dead, by definition. Over the years this teleconference has had some very wise people talk about how they try to have rituals that work for them. One year one intensive care nurse who was in the emergency room said, "Well, sex helps a lot." You just had to hug her. Honesty is a good thing.

GB: If you had just one message that you'd like to get to caregivers in particular, what would it be?

CR: There are times of acute caregiving, but caregiving is something you do and want to do all of your life, and my basic view is that we should just rejoice in it. That anyone who has ever really thought about it knows that it is by far the most rewarding thing you'll ever do.

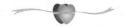

Mountains

Caregiving responsibilities consist of numerous mountains that appear first as *obstacles*. So much has to be done, learned, and changed in rapid-fire fashion that you can easily become unnerved, bewildered, or overwhelmed by the tasks set before you. The trick is to break down these tasks into small, individual steps that you can take at your own pace while still caring for your loved one.

After you develop a routine of sorts, you begin to gain a measure of confidence in your ability to make and handle crucial decisions, to rely on your own instincts rather than on sources not involved in the caregiving situation itself. In other words, little by little, you learn how to cope.

What you do not see during this process, and are usually quite oblivious to, is that each step you take creates opportunities out of those obstacles. You are gaining something positive for every negative experience you face. Often, it is only in hindsight that we truly do realize this profound truth.

Words that I penned over two decades ago, long before I ever had to actually learn from reality, much less live it, were these: "Those things placed there upon my path were meant to stumble me—but these became the steppingstones to greater victories."

The ultimate result of your caregiving? Despite the ordeals, upheavals, trials, struggles, and setbacks of the outside of you, the inside of you is becoming more resilient, sturdy, steadfast, immovable, resourceful, and self-assured. You have taken so many steps beyond where you began that, much to your own amazement, you stand atop those mountains of obstacles. Your steps led you to opportunities for growth and now you stand atop the mountain that once loomed so large and ominous in your eyes. You can see from this vantage point that you truly are an overcomer! You have weathered the storms of life on behalf of another living soul and, as a result, have found strength to override your human weakness, the inner power to withstand the buffeting of man-made opinions, and the grace to help in times of need.

You do start out at the bottom of the mountain in caregiving, where the obstacles reside. But each step you take brings opportunities for inner growth, and, ultimately, you find that those things that you thought were for the worst have turned out to be for the very best. But it is only after the caregiving is complete and you stand atop that mountain as an overcomer of all that has befallen and ensnared you that you can truly grasp this for a reality and incorporate it into your concept of yourself. It does make me wonder sometimes. If we just reached up our hand through the clouds at that altitude, could we somehow feel the touch of our loved ones as they crossed over to that other side?

— © 2000 Dorothy Womack

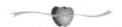

Let Us Hear from You

I invite caregivers to contact me directly with any comments or questions at gary@caregiver.com. We urge caregivers to sign up for our free online newsletter at caregiver.com. Subscriptions to *Today's Caregiver Magazine* are $18 a year and are available by calling (800) 829-2734 or by mailing payment to:

Today's Caregiver Magazine
6365 Taft Street
Suite 3006
Hollywood, Florida 33024

Index